Caesarean Birth

A positive approach to preparation and recovery

By Leigh East

First published 2011 in UK and USA by Tiskimo

Text, book design, cover design & illustrations © Leigh East

Includes: full bibliography and index

ISBN: 978-0-9568480-0-0

Keywords used in cataloguing: Birth, Caesarean, Health, Maternity,
Parenthood, Pregnancy.

A catalogue record for this book is available from the British Library.

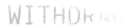

Contents

Forward

Childbirth is a hugely emotive subject and the debate about caesarean birth is particularly contentious, so much so that it can be difficult to find impartial information on this mode of birth. *Caesarean Birth – A positive approach to preparation and recovery* is possibly the first comprehensive book to bring a detailed, balanced viewpoint to this controversial subject.

As co-founder of the Birth Trauma Association, the UK charity providing support for women who have suffered traumatic experiences in childbirth, my colleagues and I see a huge amount of avoidable distress suffered by women who have received inadequate antenatal information. It is extraordinarily short-sighted to focus solely on vaginal birth and emphasise managing without pain relief. In fact, there are no guarantees and many women will not be able to achieve this. Antenatal education has a duty to help women understand that intervention, including pain relief, may be necessary and for some a caesarean will be the way their baby is delivered. Crucially it has a responsibility to show that caesarean birth can be a very positive experience and recovery just as quick as many of the less straightforward vaginal births. A much healthier approach would be to focus on a psychologically and physically healthy mother and baby rather than the means by which this is achieved.

The discourse surrounding women's choice is an interesting one and Chapter 3 *I would prefer a caesarean* is fascinating. Whilst maternally requested homebirths are increasingly gaining support from health professionals in some places, caesareans on maternal request are frequently denied unless the woman is prepared to pay for it, this despite no clear evidence that the overall risks for women planning small families are higher (see Appendix C). Women who challenge the prevailing hegemony and request caesareans are often socially stigmatised as *too posh to push* and for those women who agree to a caesarean for medical reasons, feelings of guilt and disappointment can become unnecessarily associated with the birth of their child. Antenatal education is, in general, failing women by omitting key information about caesareans when preparing them for birth. Such oppressive attitudes need to change and I see this book as a pivotal part of that change. If choice is to be respected, it needs to be informed choice and women should be given the full range of choice – from homebirth to planned caesarean.

It remains the case that childbirth is unpredictable. Relatively few women will achieve the socially defined perfect, intervention free birth (see Chapter 2) and it is tragic that they are being led to believe that they can ultimately control what happens. Such beliefs lead some women to blame themselves when things go wrong and leave others terrified when interventions like a caesarean become necessary.

This book sets the scene for what I genuinely hope will be a change in how we provide information for women antenatally. It is an invaluable handbook not only for all expectant parents but also those responsible for supporting them.

Maureen Treadwell

Co-founder of the Birth Trauma Association

Introduction

One in four women in the UK[1] (with similar figures across the developed world) experience a caesarean birth, planned or otherwise. Unplanned caesareans account for two thirds of all caesareans in the UK[2] (with similar figures elsewhere). Whether a caesarean is planned or not, the better informed you are the more flexible you are likely to be and the greater your chance of a positive experience and recovery. A positive start creates positive memories and puts you in a strong position for your adventure into motherhood.

Planned caesareans have become associated with the phrase *too posh to push*, forcing them to the periphery of antenatal education. This makes it difficult to have rational, balanced discussions about caesareans in general. Often caesareans are relegated to a few pages in birthing manuals and go little beyond the basics of anaesthetics and the number of people attending. Natural birth campaigns, while important, have portrayed caesareans as a *last resort*, leaving fear and stigma to be associated with this procedure. The result is that many women are insufficiently prepared for medical intervention and caesareans in particular.

A vaginal birth is a wonderful experience for many women. However, births do not always go to plan and medical interventions can leave some women feeling ashamed, cheated and/or intensely disappointed. Some feel they experienced an unnecessary caesarean, while others who would prefer a caesarean are denied the choice or are made to feel it is a selfish one. Some of these women easily come to terms with their births whilst others struggle.

This book has been written to help you make informed decisions about your birth. Having more information about the impact of these decisions will help you feel more confident when preparing, experiencing and recovering from your birth. It is not my intention to direct you towards a planned caesarean, or to advocate against one, but rather to provide information and ideas to make it possible for a caesarean birth to feel rewarding and fulfilling, should you have one.

While this book concentrates on making the most of a caesarean birth, many of the ideas can be used to help you recover from vaginal birth too, whether trauma has arisen from medical intervention or not. Managing to *feel* in control of your birth can dramatically improve your emotional response to it.

Using this book

It is not always possible to avoid medical jargon so there is a comprehensive glossary in an appendix. Caesarean terminology in particular differs between hospitals and countries, in this book a single set of terms will be used throughout (see Chapter 1).

The book uses the latest international research but refers to intervention and outcome rates from the UK to avoid long lists of figures from around the world. If you are birthing outside the UK check the rates for your specific country and hospital.

A great deal of care has been taken in the researching and writing of this book, however, it should not be used in isolation. Your pregnancy is specific to you and you should seek medical advice regarding it. This book provides you with medical information to help you in those discussions.

About the author

I experienced first-hand the difficulties of researching an unpopular birth mode and the pressure exerted when planning a caesarean with and without a recognised medical need.

I witnessed a traumatic birth at the age of 19 in a Romanian hospital but was unaware of the real impact this had until I became pregnant myself. This upsetting experience coupled with various birth stories of my friends' unplanned caesareans made me realise I needed to know more about what I might be facing. Of 13 friends already with children, 7 had had unplanned caesareans, all had been very frightened and some severely traumatised by the experience. My initial research focused on finding out more about caesarean birth and how to avoid it, a difficult task in itself as most birth books dedicate only a couple of pages to caesareans. As I talked to more and more mothers, including some doctors themselves planning a caesarean in the absence of currently accepted medical needs, I came to realise that there was a lot more to it than just waiting to see what happened on the day.

Following the birth of my first daughter after a planned caesarean at 39.4 weeks I created _csections.org_ to share my research with others. The website now has over 2000 unique visitors a month. My second daughter was another planned caesarean though she decided to come early and after 8 hours of early labour she was born by caesarean at 38.3 weeks. Both births were thrilling, I held my babies in theatre and tried feeding them in the recovery room. While I found walking uncomfortable for the first few days there have been no lasting effects and I exclusively breastfed both girls, only stopping when they decided it was time.

For me planned caesareans were the right choice. Following the development of _csections.org_ I began working closely with several organisations and co-founded *coalitionforchildbirthautonomy.org*. Together we campaign for *accurate* information and support for women in childbirth. We help to bring about change through stakeholder involvement on the UK NICE Guideline on Caesarean Birth and as user representatives on the UK Government Working Party for Maternity Care.

I am a mum not a doctor. A wonderful network of specialists have participated in the development of this book (see Acknowledgements), but the final text remains my opinion and responsibility. I am confident everything you read is accurate and based on up-to-date research.

CHAPTER ONE

Caesareans explained

What is a caesarean?

A caesarean is the delivery of your baby through a surgical cut in your abdomen and uterus. It is most frequently used when a vaginal birth is perceived to carry greater risk than a surgical delivery, for either you or your baby. It may be planned ahead of labour or its need identified as labour progresses.

A caesarean is a surgical event whereas a vaginal birth is hopefully, primarily a biological one. There are obvious differences in terms of the physical experience but emotionally the differences are less clear. Emotional highs and lows can follow both modes of birth.

Terminology

There are many phrases associated with caesareans. Most have emotional baggage: *life-saving, last resort, scary,* even *selfish.* Terms are used inconsistently making it all rather confusing.

The most common terms are:

- **Planned, Scheduled and Elective** – These are pre-arranged caesareans. You may have requested the caesarean or had it recommended by a practitioner and labour has not usually begun. The term elective has become an emotive one often used in the *too posh to push* debate

- **Emergency, Unplanned, Critical and Crash** – These refer to situations where a vaginal birth is planned but events have taken over before or during labour and your baby is delivered by caesarean

The terms *planned* and *unplanned* will be used throughout this book.

Planned caesarean

These are agreed in advance and occur prior to labour unless specifically requested. Typically they follow a practitioner's recommendation but may have been at your suggestion.

Planned caesareans usually happen in week 39 (weeks 37-8 for multiple births). If you would prefer labour to start the process, check the safety of this for your specific situation. Of course your baby may have other ideas and come early. Approximately 1 in 10 women go into labour before their planned caesarean.[5]

A planned caesarean *should* be calm and you will have had opportunity to discuss the caesarean before the day. Your situation is well documented and on the day each step can be explained to you with no need to rush. Many aspects of a caesarean birth plan can be accommodated (see Chapter 5).

Natural caesarean

A planned, *natural* caesarean is a new development used by a few UK practitioners for straightforward pregnancies (not available for breech or transverse babies).[6] [7] The overall experience is calm and personalised and includes:

- Delivery of her head first

- Delivery paused to support acclimatisation, taking her first breaths while her body is still in the womb (compression may help expel fluid from her lungs)

- Delayed cord cutting (2 minutes) until breathing has stabilised

- Lights dimmed on delivery

- Screen lowered on delivery so you can see her lifted from you and you can determine the sex

- Immediate skin-to-skin contact as she is delivered onto your chest (ECG wires are attached to your back rather than your chest) where she is covered and positioned so you can try breastfeeding

---

To labour or not to labour

Waiting to go into labour before your caesarean might be a good way of ensuring your baby is dictating her arrival time thereby possibly reducing the risk of respiratory distress. With any luck she will start things off close to week 40, have good lung maturity and benefit from hormonal changes triggered during birth. However, caesareans conducted during labour carry some increased risks, such that many hospitals classify them as emergencies. Increased risks are: surgical nicks to your baby[3], infection[4] and difficulty inserting needles (where contractions are close together). There is also no guarantee that staff and theatres will be available when you decide you are ready for your caesarean.

Natural caesarean

This calm, gentle approach can accommodate many of your birth preferences and "pausing [surgery with only the head delivered] allows external compression from the uterus and maternal soft tissues to expel lung liquid." Professor Nicholas Fisk, Consultant Obstetrician & Gynaecologist[8] et al

Unplanned caesarean

There are two types of unplanned caesarean and in both, labour may or may not have begun when events occur making it necessary to deliver your baby *soon* (see Appendix B):

Emergency caesarean

A vaginal birth was planned but complications arising during pregnancy or labour, while not immediately life-threatening, mean you and your baby would benefit from early delivery. If an epidural is already in place this will be used to administer the anaesthetic – one will be inserted if not. Regional anaesthesia is used wherever possible so you are awake.

> *A mum referring to her planned caesarean after a previous unplanned one said "I was absolutely exhausted after my first caesarean. I laboured for over 25 hours and was so frightened by the emergency, this was a walk in the park by comparison." Natalie (32)*

Critical caesarean

A situation has arisen during your pregnancy or labour meaning it is essential your baby be delivered as soon as possible. The situation may require a general anaesthetic as it is the fastest way of administering your pain relief and delivering your baby safely.[9]

How do planned and unplanned caesareans differ?

Full details of the procedure are elsewhere (see Chapter 1 & Appendix A).

Practical differences

- In an emergency events move quickly, it can feel chaotic and frightening. Set-up for planned caesareans is slower and everything is explained to you

- In an emergency you may get little notice that a caesarean is needed, whereas you may have had weeks or months to prepare for a planned caesarean

> *A mother who signed a consent form prior to an unplanned caesarean during a protracted labour said "I did not have time to read anything. I was just grateful someone was helping me, but as a lawyer I worried afterwards that I had signed something without reading it." Angela (33)*

- Unplanned caesareans often come at the end of hours of labour so you are likely to be exhausted. With your planned caesarean unless you are waiting for signs of labour, you should be fresh and alert going into theatre

- With a planned caesarean you are less likely to experience labour unless you have arranged to wait for it

- *Critical* caesareans may use general anaesthetic, which means not only will you be asleep during delivery but you are likely to be drowsy afterwards making you and your baby disinterested or unable to feed for several hours. Planned caesareans typically use regional anaesthetics which do not cause drowsiness

Emotional differences

Emotionally the difference between a planned and unplanned caesarean can feel substantial. This is dependent partly upon the circumstances leading to surgery but also upon how prepared you were for such a possibility arising. In addition:

> *A mum referring to her unplanned caesarean said "I found it really frightening and my husband was shoved out of the room. I was so exhausted I do not remember anything other than being terrified."*
> *Becky (33)*

- The rapid changes of an unplanned caesarean can be frightening. You may be anxious about a planned caesarean too but will have had time to prepare and ask questions

- After a long labour you may feel disheartened your birth is ending with an unplanned caesarean. Some mums are relieved, others traumatised by the radical deviation from their vaginal birth plan, reporting feelings of distress and failure

- An unplanned caesarean may require a general anaesthetic resulting in hours passing before you hold your baby. Some women feel this delay affects their ability to bond with their baby

- Breastfeeding may be adversely affected or delayed after an unplanned caesarean due to a combination of distress, exhaustion, physical discomfort or general anaesthetic

Perception of suffering

In a survey asking mums if they thought they had *suffered* as a result of their caesarean, over 60% said they did not. Of those having a planned caesarean 80% felt they had not suffered compared to 55% of those experiencing an unplanned one.[10]

Depressed thoughts and negative feelings are unfortunately quite common after unplanned caesareans and some women do feel disappointed they have not given birth vaginally. There are several things you can do to help reduce severe negative reactions (see Chapter 5) and improve your recovery (see Chapter 6).

Risk differences

There are risks associated with caesareans that increase during unplanned caesareans:

- While slight, there is an increased risk of surgical injury to you and your baby due to: the speed of an unplanned delivery, the reason for the caesarean and whether or not you are already in labour

> A mum talking about a planned caesarean after an unplanned one said "It was entirely different, all the things you hope your birth will be: calm, peaceful, relaxed. This beginning with W was so much better, we bonded more and I could feed him. I wasn't at all exhausted." Meg (37)

- If all attempts at vaginal delivery have been made (e.g. forceps) you will be very tired and may experience *damage* to your vaginal area

What are my anaesthetic options?

You will be offered one of the following:

- Spinal (regional)
- Epidural (regional)
- Combined spinal and epidural (regional)
- General

The following is a brief summary of each. Your hospital must make sure you understand your options[11] as you will be asked to consent to the type used. You may want have such a discussion even when planning a vaginal birth as you may request an epidural during labour. A third of UK women end up having one of the following during birth: epidural, spinal or general anaesthetic.[12]

You should aim to understand:

- The benefits and risks of each
- Which is best suited to your specific circumstances
- Which options your hospital offer

Regional anaesthetic

A regional anaesthetic numbs a specific part of your body so you can be awake throughout surgery.

There are three types: epidural, spinal and combined spinal/epidural. There are subtle differences between them and it is *very* important to discuss these with an anaesthetist. The following is a simplified description:

- **Epidural** – Administered through a fine tube in your back which remains in place throughout surgery. It is topped up as needed and takes effect within 20 minutes

- **Spinal** – A single injection to your lower back. It is quicker, easier, less painful to administer and uses a lower dose with a more dense block than an epidural[13] but it cannot be topped up (it lasts at least 1.5-2 hours, much longer than most caesareans)

- **Combined spinal / epidural** – A combination of the above starting with a smaller dose of spinal topped up using the epidural tube as needed

General anaesthetic

A general anaesthetic acts on your brain, putting you completely to sleep. It is very fast acting (within 5 minutes) and your caesarean can then be performed very quickly. It is administered through an intravenous tube (IV) and you will be asked to breathe oxygen through a facemask before you go to sleep.

It does carry a greater degree of risk than regional anaesthetic (see Appendix C) but is only used where surgery needs to be carried out as quickly as possible, where other forms of anaesthesia are not working or where the anaesthetist deems the balance of risk indicates a general is more advantageous e.g. serious bleeding or infection etc.

What are the benefits and risks of caesarean and vaginal birth?

Vaginal birth is a wonderful and natural process with many benefits for both you and your baby, but it has risks and is an experience over which you only have a certain amount of control. That said caesareans should not be viewed as an easier option, they

> *"Going through the pain and jubilation of labour and birth gives us an empathic understanding of what our baby has just been through."*
> *Holly 35*

carry significant risks too. So while hoping everything goes according to your plan, try not to base your assessment of benefits/risks on the idea that certain things just will not happen to you.

As you read this book or any other material on this subject, ensure you make reasonable comparisons. Compare like for like e.g. a planned caesarean with a planned vaginal birth. Do not be tempted to compare a straightforward, natural vaginal birth with a *critical* caesarean. The latter is a possible outcome of the former.

Evaluating risks is difficult. Some risks are the same whichever way you give birth, others are very different and it is all a matter of personal opinion as to which risks feel more significant.

If you are in a position to decide whether you have a vaginal birth or a caesarean, think about your personal circumstances and how these might alter your level of risk. For example, if you are over weight or obese there is an increased likelihood of your birth ending as a caesarean regardless of how straightforward your pregnancy has been (see Appendix C). If you are planning on having a large family then be aware that the risk of developing certain medical conditions increases with the number of caesareans you have (see Appendix C).

> **Informed choice**
>
> "The risks of CS [caesarean section] and labour are real but different and if fully explained to the woman, she should be allowed to accept one set of risks over the other – after all she is the person who has to live with the consequences." Sara Paterson -Brown, Consultant Obstetrician, Queen Charlotte's & Chelsea Hospital, London [14]

For a full list of the benefits and risks of both vaginal and caesarean birth see Appendix C. Bear in mind that this list includes all risks, even those that are extremely rare, so it may feel rather long and daunting.

CHAPTER TWO

Why prepare for a caesarean birth?

Caesareans are a possible outcome of every birth. Making plans with this in mind improves your flexibility, an important factor in how you view the whole experience. A survey comparing birth perceptions of women that were *informed* (or not) about caesareans prior to birth found that 7 in 100 *informed* women perceived their caesarean as traumatic compared with 35 in 100 of those who had not prepared.[15]

Why prepare?

By preparing you stand a very good chance of:

- Influencing what happens before, during and after your birth
- Increasing the level of involvement you and your birth partner have in your birth
- Negotiating effectively in situations where a caesarean is still only a recommendation
- Reducing the likelihood of subsequent emotional distress
- Improving your overall recovery experience
- Avoiding unnecessary intervention

What should I know?

Why a caesarean might be recommended

Understanding the reasons why caesareans are sometimes suggested means you can engage in positive discussion in a calm and informed manner. Knowing when they are *necessary* or just a matter of opinion, you can decide how much importance to attach to a recommendation (see Appendix B).

> *"I was totally unprepared for my first experience of birth. It was quite scary and I really knew very little about induction or caesarean birth before experiencing them. I felt very stressed throughout the whole procedure." Anna (31)*

What the caesarean might be like

Some women prefer not to know details, others feel more confident if they know as much as possible. However, there are several points in a caesarean where you can significantly influence your experience. Knowing this can inform your birth plan and in an unplanned caesarean help you make choices more quickly and confidently (see Chapter 5 & Appendix A).

> **Origins of birth dis-satisfaction**
>
> A survey of more than 250 mums who experienced a caesarean found that "much of the dissatisfaction among the emergency caesarean group stemmed from their lack of preparation for an operative delivery" Dr Colin Francome, Emeritus Professor in the Sociology of Health at Middlesex University[16] et al

What your rights are

It may help to know your rights, particularly if you experience conflict over your birth preference. Never be afraid to ask questions. Keep asking until you fully understand why a caesarean is being recommended (or refused) (see Chapter 4).

What the keys things to learn might be

While you have time, learn about the procedure and how to prepare yourself, your home and your family as well as how to support your recovery. If you are hoping to avoid a caesarean, try not to ignore that it is a possibility. Research suggests that you are at increased risk of a negative reaction to medical intervention if you have not been prepared for this possibility antenatally.[18]

If you are hoping to have one, you may find discussions take several appointments. If your request is unsuccessful you may need time to come to terms with and plan for a vaginal birth or find a more willing practitioner (see Chapter 3).

> **Failure to progress**
>
> The stalling of labour, also referred to as *failure to progress* is thought to currently account for 25% of caesareans.[17] However on its own, it is not a reason to agree to a caesarean if you would rather continue to labour.

How flexible to be

Many mums develop views about the way they want their birth to go. Do have a preference, but it should be just that – a preference. Things change, both your circumstances and your perceptions. A safe delivery should be the driving factor. [More info.[i]]

The more rigid your views, the more likely you are to experience feelings ranging from disappointment or distress to full post-traumatic stress

---

[i] www.askamum.co.uk search for Are natural childbirth classes a waste of time?

disorder, if you are unable to achieve your goals.[19] You can help reduce the impact of unplanned interventions by having the knowledge to discuss what happens next (see Chapter 5 & Appendix A). Try to view a caesarean not as a failure of your body or of those caring for you, but simply as another route to the safe delivery of your baby.

Manage your expectations

The big picture

The UK caesarean rate is 1 in 4[21], (1 in 3 in the US[22]) with similar figures elsewhere in the developed world. Despite media coverage to the contrary there is no clear evidence for an ideal target rate and the World Health Organisation has retracted its previous recommendations on this.[23]

More than 50% of UK births involve intervention (epidural, instruments, induction or caesarean)[24] and a third of women have either an epidural, spinal or general anaesthetic at some point in their birth.[25] A UK survey found only 10% of women achieve a totally natural birth[26] (1% in the US[27]).

In the last few decades there have been significant improvements in the techniques, experience and outcome of caesareans. It is safer than before but *not* risk free, easier or better than a straightforward vaginal birth. There are risks with both (see Appendix C).

Both vaginal birth and caesarean recovery are painful but effective pain relief can mitigate pain. However UK figures[28] suggest nearly half of women attending antenatal classes are encouraged to avoid pain relief for vaginal birth even though three quarters report labour was "more painful than they ever imagined" (Mother and Baby survey 2005[29]). Bear in mind too that the average delay in obtaining pain relief after requesting an epidural is 60 minutes.

Origins of preferences

"Choices that are made throughout labour are made on the basis of how women anticipate labour pain. For example, if a woman views labour as a medical condition with risks, she may be more likely to choose pain relief to eradicate the pain. If, however, she views labour as a normal and natural process, she may be more likely to employ natural methods of coping with pain relief." Joanne E Lally, Research Fellow at Institute of Health and Society, Newcastle University[20] et al

It is important therefore that while you can and should develop preferences you should also attempt to understand the origins of your preferences and evaluate the reality your approach may lead to.

Despite recommendations to the contrary almost two thirds of UK women[30] lie in bed unnecessarily for much of their labour. They may be attached to fetal monitors for significant periods if there are concerns about the baby. The average first time mum still spends 3 days in hospital because of various complications associated with delivery, whether or not she gave birth vaginally.[31] Totally *natural* births can be quite difficult to achieve.

Check the facts

Many myths about caesareans abound and the media perpetuate these. Information is often presented as fact but only by reading the original research can you discover the full truth.

Common myths:

Caesareans will cause respiratory problems for your baby

Media reviews of studies fail to clarify that the risk of breathing problems in babies born at 39 weeks or later is very low and not statistically significantly different from babies born vaginally at the same gestational stage (see Appendix C). Nor do they mention that health guidelines recommend caesareans before 39 weeks should only be done if there are important medical reasons. Whilst it is the case that being born before this can cause respiratory problems for *some* babies, early caesareans (pre 38 weeks) are usually necessary for other medical reasons and such media scaremongering only serves to increase the fear and guilt for those women who need an early caesarean.

7.3%[32] (73 in 1,000) of women are *too posh to push*

This frequently misused figure is often cited in the *elective* caesarean debate. Yet it actually incorporates *all* maternally requested caesareans including those which follow recommendations from the mother's practitioner, i.e. when medical situations indicate that a caesarean might be necessary.[34] [35] The actual number is thought to be much lower and include those women with tokophobia (fear of childbirth), previous traumatic births and abuse. In other words a judgemental statement like *too posh to push* entirely misses the complexity of women's decision-making and takes no account of the discrepancy in the coding of births that can occur between hospitals[36] (see Appendix B).

> "So maybe we should stop judging the elective (or non-elective) C-section mothers, or feeling guilty for not having vaginal births, or developing inferiority complexes because we broke down and got an epidural. Maybe we should realise that the test of our motherhood really begins once that healthy child arrives on this Earth and in our arms."
> Jenny Chaney, journalist at the Washington Post[33]

Caesareans carry significantly higher risks than vaginal delivery

Research is often compromised by combining unplanned (caesareans carried out as a result of a medical emergency) and planned caesareans (those conducted with known medical situations or no medical need) into a single statistic and by poor documentation of intended mode of birth.[37] [38]

The two procedures are actually very different, carrying different levels of risk (see Chapter 1 & Appendix C).[39] A Swedish study reveals that, when the two types of caesarean are separated, the death rates for vaginal birth and planned caesarean are very low and almost identical (5 and 4 in 10,000 respectively) and only unplanned caesareans show a higher rate of risk (29 in 10,000).[40]

Prepare in advance

There are lots of things you can do to prepare for a caesarean. Planning means that if a caesarean does happen you are in the best possible position to make the most of it. You may like to consider the following:

- **Write a birth plan** – You can express a preference on specific aspects of your surgery as well as the details of your baby's first experiences outside the womb. You can also express preferences about the sort of things you would prefer to avoid (see Chapter 5). The more things you think about in advance the less there is to negotiate on the day

- **Prepare for an extended stay in hospital** – You will be in hospital for 2-3 days minimum, though some women, with good home support, can go home sooner (see Chapter 5)

- **Develop new skills** – Learn alternative breastfeeding positions to make feeding more comfortable following surgery (see Chapter 5 & Chapter 6)

- **Prepare your home and family** – You will need more support in the first couple of weeks. This is often true of women who have a vaginal delivery, but in the case of a caesarean birth you *know* you will need help so plan for it (see Chapter 5)

Make realistic comparisons

Clarify the information you are given. Women are frequently told caesareans carry a higher level of risk. When grouped together, planned and unplanned caesareans do carry higher risk of death than vaginal birth. However "when you consider only [planned] caesareans involving epidural analgesia, death rates are actually lower than the mortality rates associated with *all* vaginal births." Maureen Connolly, Birth Commentator [41] et al

Planned and unplanned caesareans are not the same (see Chapter 1 & Appendix C) and should not be grouped together when attempting to assess levels of risk. An emergency caesarean is typically an outcome of a vaginal birth attempt or underlying medical condition.

"Women who request caesareans are *not* requesting emergency caesareans." Maureen Treadwell, Co-founder of the Birth Trauma Association.

CHAPTER THREE

I would prefer a caesarean

Understanding your reason for wanting a caesarean is a crucial part of your preparation. It is not the most common birth choice, nor the most accepted. A request may be treated with suspicion by those who do not understand it. Some hospitals and practitioners support caesarean delivery on maternal request (CDMR), some do not. In many countries a caesarean is not an automatic right, so statements about *human rights* and *freedom of choice* are not enough. Where CDMR is not supported a hospital can refuse your request but should refer you for a second opinion.

With this in mind, approach discussions as knowledgeably and rationally as you can.

Understanding your preference

Use facts as well as feelings to explain your reason. The way you present them can make all the difference to how your request is received.

For example, concern that a vaginal birth will affect your sex life is unlikely to be accepted if you are healthy, except in the context of a psychological condition such as vaginismus (where the pelvic floor muscles and vagina can involuntarily tighten) or prior trauma caused by sexual abuse.

Combining your reasons may prove more effective. Preferences based on safety or control, are very much down to an individual's personal opinion and perspective of risk, therefore it is difficult to negotiate on this basis alone.

Things to do

Before making your request, think about the following:

- **Understand your reason** – Is it based on a recognised medical condition? (see Appendix B)

- **Research your options** – Have you fully explored vaginal birth? Following which make sure you understand:

  - The difference between a planned and an unplanned caesarean (see Chapter 1)

- The risks and benefits of a caesarean, for both you and your baby (see Appendix C)

- The implications of caesareans on future pregnancies (see Appendix C)

- **Gain support** – Is your birth partner supportive? Does your hospital have specific policies regarding caesareans and do they support CDMR?

- **Define your expectations** – Make sure you understand:

  - What is important to you about your birth? (see Chapter 5)

  - What size family you are hoping to have? (see Chapter 4)

- **Question your practitioners** – Practitioners witness labour and birth regularly and it is easy to forget how a first time mother can feel. Do not let this put you off asking questions but avoid a combative approach (see Appendix F)

- **Talk to mothers** – Particularly those who have given birth in your chosen hospital or birth unit. Women naturally feel very strongly about their birth experience, good or bad, so these may be emotional stories, but think about what you can learn from them. Assess them on the basis of:

  - How recent their experience was (practices even 5 years ago may differ radically from today)

  - The amount of support they had before, during and after their experience

  - Were they open minded about the course their birth may take (e.g. if they hoped for a water birth at home but ended up being rushed into hospital their perceptions of their birth could be very negative)

- **Visit the hospital/birthing unit** – Most places offer tours to expectant parents. It is not always possible to visit an operating theatre or special care unit (SCU) but you might want to ask questions about what facilities there are (see Appendix F)

- **Assess your hospital** – Statistics should be available from the hospital itself as well as national surveys or official bodies covering: caesarean rates, other forms of intervention, VBAC (Vaginal Birth After Caesarean) rates, anaesthetic preference etc. Request their childbirth policy documents to give you an idea of specific procedural policies

- **Involve your birth partner in this process** – Discuss your reasons for preferring a caesarean. Your birth partner is likely to have worries and questions too. They play a significant part in your birth before, during and after (see Chapter 7) and can make the whole experience a lot easier

Requesting a caesarean

Talk openly with your midwife or doctor. If agreement is given at this stage ensure it is documented then make an appointment with your consultant. Detailed discussion of your birth will probably not begin until around week 30 when you can discuss the procedure, decide the type of anaesthetic and agree on the delivery date etc.

If your midwife does not agree you need to be referred to another practitioner to discuss your specific case. The practitioner may agree at this stage and the process outlined above begins. If this does not happen you need to keep going round this loop, planning your approach with care. UK hospitals cannot refuse your request without referring you for a second opinion.[43] Of course this second opinion may also refuse if they believe the caesarean is really not in the best interests of you or your baby.

In countries where you can choose your practitioner, talk specifically about caesarean options from the outset. If you pay for healthcare check your insurance company will support CDMR if there are no medical reasons for your request.

> ## Be open and honest
>
> Be as open as you can with your practitioners. Without all relevant information it is difficult for them to support you in your decision-making. "Sometimes there may be reasons for wanting a CS [caesarean] that are important to the woman but not apparent to healthcare professionals...Women could have deep-seated fears of birth, which they may be reluctant to share with healthcare professionals." Jane Weaver, Researcher from the Centre for Family Research, University of Cambridge [42] et al

Presenting your case

In the meeting itself:

- Stick to the facts (have them written down so you do not go blank) and refer to them openly. This shows you are organised and mean what you say

- Keep your tone reasonable

- Keep your points rational and factual

- Take someone with you, preferably your birth partner, both to support you but also to help you maintain perspective during discussions, (they could also take notes)

Help, they will not listen!

Try not to panic. Try to understand the reasons being given. It may be the hospital policy does not support CDMR or perhaps the person you are speaking to cannot make the decision.

If you are getting nowhere try not to get upset, finish the appointment and make the next one with a different practitioner. This may simply be another midwife/obstetrician at your local surgery/hospital or it may require a referral to another hospital.

> **A duty of care**
>
> The UK General Medical Council states that it is the duty of clinicians "to recognise that even when active treatment is not indicated, the duty to provide care to alleviate distress remains."[44] In other words, in cases of tokophobia for example it may be possible to justify a caesarean on the grounds of extreme distress.

Your rights

The patient support group in your hospital should be able to point you to documents or governing bodies that manage the standardisation of patient care. There should be documentation relating specifically to maternity care.

The following is based on the UK:

- Your practitioners must answer any questions you have about *all* birth options before you commit to anything.[45] They should clarify why a particular approach is being suggested, what will happen, the risks and benefits associated, any alternatives and their associated risks. You must then formally accept or reject the advice and sign the appropriate form[46] [More info.[ii]]

- You can request a second opinion on any matter relating to your maternity care.[47] [48] In the case of CDMR or refusing a caesarean recommendation your practitioner is obliged to agree to a referral. Referral may be to a colleague within the hospital, another NHS hospital or a privately funded hospital

> **UK rights**
>
> In the UK a caesarean is not a right but a flat refusal is difficult without a supporting policy from the hospital. If you have different opinions about your birth your practitioner should, at the very least, refer you for a second opinion.

- You can access counselling to deal with childbirth related issues e.g. severe fear of childbirth – tokophobia (this may be required before a CDMR will be considered in any case)[49]

[ii] www.rcog.org.uk search for Consent Advice no. 7 Caesarean Birth

- You can ask to see your medical notes at any time, whether you are having your appointments at hospital or in your local doctor's surgery[50]

- Your consent must have been received (in writing) before surgery can be carried out. You still have the right to change your mind, though this too should be documented. In the case of an unplanned caesarean where timing is critical, oral consent will suffice[51]

- You can refuse a course of action that is being recommended to you (informed refusal). You may be required to sign documentation to this effect.

If you plan a vaginal birth it is still helpful to know your rights. Circumstances can quickly change during labour. Pain and tiredness can make it difficult to discuss things that are entirely new to you. Understanding your rights will help you feel more confident in your subsequent decisions. Knowing you were able to fully engage in informed debate may help you cope emotionally after your birth if it does not go to plan.

Going elsewhere

If you end up changing hospitals there are a few things to bear in mind before making a final decision:

> **Human rights**
>
> The UK has been a signatory to the European Convention on Human Rights (ECHR) for more than 50 years. Since 1998 the UK's Human Rights Act has meant that the UK has a legal as well as moral obligation to conform to the principles of the (ECHR). Article 3 is particularly pertinent to childbirth and refers to freedom from torture, inhuman and degrading treatment. Case law shows that "Neglectful failure to provide the care which is necessary to avoid preventable suffering can amount to inhuman or degrading treatment." Emmanuel Kant, Barrister[52]

- **Policy statements** – Check their childbirth policies. Some hospitals aim to reduce the caesarean rate and/or refuse CDMR. If your situation does not require a caesarean there is little point investigating birth at such a hospital. Many of those that offer CDMR will still state that agreement will be given on the condition that the planned caesarean does not put you at significant risk. It will be up to you to determine what they mean by *significant risk* and to negotiate around this. Some hospitals leave decision-making entirely to individual practitioners

- **Statistics** – Understand rates of intervention and preferred practice. Information should be available from the hospital. Some may appear to have lower rates of intervention because they only accept low risk pregnancies. If you are in a particular situation (e.g. multiple births, breech etc.), make sure they are experienced in dealing with this. Conversely, a hospital specialising in specific types of complex birth may *appear* to a have higher caesarean rate

- **Hospital size** – Smaller hospitals may not have a SCU. Bear in mind you could find yourself separated (i.e. in a different hospital) from your baby if one of you requires extra help

- **Additional costs** – There may be a substantial difference in fees, particularly in the UK where NHS hospitals do not have any fees (unless you request a private room), but private hospitals do and many health insurers no longer cover CDMR. In the case of alternative UK NHS hospitals, travel costs are likely to be the only additional expense

> **Respecting informed choice**
>
> "We should respect a woman's view and choice if it is fully informed, if she expresses a logical reason for wanting a caesarean section, and if she can demonstrate an understanding of the implications of the procedure. We should not be dictating to women what they should think, nor should we be judgmental of their values if they happen to differ from our own." Sara Paterson-Brown, Consultant Obstetrician, Queen Charlotte's and Chelsea Hospital, London[53]

- **Accessibility** – The alternative hospital may be further away. This is important not only for getting there in time should your baby decide to arrive early, but also for birth partners and siblings to visit, particularly where there is a prolonged hospital stay

They have agreed, what next?

First make sure the agreement is documented in your medical notes, then:

- Plan the details of your birth (see Appendix E)

- Prepare your body, your home, your friends/family and your children for the arrival of your baby (see Chapter 5)

What if I go into labour early?

Your plans may sometimes need to alter. Your baby may decide to come early or your pregnancy may suddenly change requiring intervention. If you have a caesarean agreed this should still go ahead. However, in such cases there may be delays, theatres may be busy, appropriate staff unavailable or you may be unable to reach hospital quickly. There are a number of things that you can do to help prepare for this:

- **Learn coping techniques** – Techniques used to help women prepare for vaginal delivery, such as breathing, relaxation, meditation and massage, will be equally valuable in keeping you calm during the early stages of labour

- **Access counselling** – Get help in advance with fears surrounding childbirth. Your practitioners should have a list of counsellors

- **Employ additional support** – This can be pricey, but if it is possible you could consider a doula or independent midwife. She can work with you during your pregnancy then accompany you throughout your birth, whether it is a planned caesarean or a vaginal birth, though once in hospital she will not have the power to overrule decisions made by hospital staff

- **Research vaginal delivery** – The more knowledge you have of labour and vaginal birth, the more confident you may feel should you labour for longer than expected or indeed deliver vaginally. Attend birth classes even if you are planning a caesarean and look at other resources, books, videos and classes (see Other resources)

Coping with disapproval

Whatever decision you make about how you would prefer to give birth, you will find someone who has a different opinion.

Comments come from the most unusual places including employers, friends (male as well as female) and perhaps most surprisingly from people who have no experience of childbirth. Opinions can vary and you should not be surprised if you have at least one very uncomfortable conversation either before or after your caesarean.

Responding to typical challenges

It will be necessary to engage in difficult discussions with your practitioners particularly if your request runs counter to their advice. However, with family, friends and colleagues, it is really up to you how much debate you get into.

If you can, look at the situation objectively and determine whether you really care what the other person thinks. If the answer is no, then walk away, confident in your *informed* decision. There is no need to be confrontational. Something along the lines of "what is right for one person is not always right for another" will get you off the hook in many situations.

If you do care about their opinion and want to debate or justify your decision it is worth having answers for the most common questions and challenges you are likely to face. There are many myths surrounding caesareans and being aware of these and knowing the facts will be helpful (see Chapter 1, Appendix B & Appendix C).

If you have medical reasons you are prepared to talk about you may find it easier to justify your decision, referring to your caesarean as *recommended* rather than *planned* or *elective*. Where your reasons are more personal or *non-standard* it is worth thinking about whether or not you want to divulge them. For example, it may not be appropriate to share feelings of intense fear with another pregnant woman. If your reasons may not be considered socially acceptable, for example, planning a caesarean so you can manage work commitments, think about whether you really want to get into a debate about it. Similarly if your reason is the result of abuse, previous trauma or a current medical condition (yours or your baby's) it may be too painful to discuss.

> *"She [the consultant] raised her eyebrows and rolled her eyes at the nurse. I had gone in thinking I had already been told I had to have a caesarean after last time and she was treating me as if I was too posh to push. She clearly hadn't read my notes. I had CPD, [Cephalo Pelvic Disproportion] and when she realised that she changed her tune but I felt really depressed after seeing her."* Anne (27)

Ultimately the reasons are personal to you and you do not need to justify your preference to anyone other than your practitioner and birth partner. A belligerent "because I want one" may be enough in your view but may not reassure your parents or best-friend who probably just wants to make sure you know what you are doing.

It is also worth bearing in mind that even if you have an unplanned caesarean you may still hear surprising comments. These tend to revolve around assumptions that you are disappointed or that you did not birth *properly*, or that subsequent problems are to be directly blamed on the caesarean. Certainly some women do feel traumatised as a result of having not given birth *properly* (see Chapter 6) but this is not the case for everyone and it can be hurtful to have such assumptions made. Whether your caesarean is planned or not try not to worry about the opinions of others.

CHAPTER FOUR

I do not want a caesarean

The act of giving birth is, for many women, a fulfilling and important part of becoming a parent. This natural, physiological process plays an important part in ensuring your baby is ready for birth and the outside world. Many women prefer to let labour unfold naturally and with good preparation and support this is possible for a significant number. If you would rather avoid a caesarean it is important you know what factors can increase their likelihood and what conditions require a caesarean. Unfortunately there are cases where women feel their caesarean was unnecessary, but with knowledge you can help manage your birth, distinguishing those situations where a caesarean really is the only option from those where you can still labour.

What are the most common reasons given for needing a caesarean?

The most common reasons for a caesarean being recommended are:

- Previous caesarean
- Failure to progress
- Breech lying baby
- Distress of mum and/or baby

However, in *all* these cases it is actually still a matter of opinion and individual circumstances (see Appendix B).

What can I do to reduce the chance of having a caesarean?

Avoiding a caesarean needs the same research and knowledge as requesting one, particularly if your situation is not straightforward (see Appendix C).

Be informed

Clarify why a caesarean is being recommended, particularly what benefits you can expect over a vaginal birth. If necessary ask for assistance in evaluating the risks in your specific circumstances, this may involve a second opinion.

Check if there are any other options open to you e.g. trying to turn your baby if the caesarean is recommended for a breech.

Understand which practices are linked with unplanned caesareans. A phenomenon referred to as *cascade of intervention* is believed to contribute. For example, induction and the use of fetal heart monitors – which reduce mobility and increase time spent lying on your back – can have a knock-on effect on your ability to labour effectively[54] setting off a chain of events that may result in *failure to progress*. This diagnosis can, if unchallenged result in a caesarean (see Appendix B).

Know your rights (see Chapter 3). Calmly discussing your options, knowing what can and cannot be insisted upon and the difference between a *required* and *suggested* caesarean, puts you in a strong negotiating position. For example, if your baby is lying with her spine to your spine (posterior position), she has further to turn before birth and this can significantly extend the duration of your labour. Knowing this means that *failing to progress* may actually just be a longer labour because of her position. A recent study showed that waiting for 2 hours following the point at which the cervix has been identified as *stalled* during active labour can result in a third of women still achieving a vaginal birth.[56]

> **Understand your rights**
>
> "English law supports the right of a competent individual to decline treatment (a *negative* right)" Leonie Penna, Consultant obstetrician, Kings College Hospital, London.[55] US case law appears to extend much greater rights to the fetus.

Create a birth plan

Certain decisions *may* reduce the likelihood of medical intervention including an unplanned caesarean (e.g. not having continuous fetal monitoring[57] [58] or labouring at home for as long as possible), so developing a birth plan with these preferences may make a difference.

In addition, a birth plan incorporating your preferences in the event of a caesarean will help guide practitioners and improve your experience (see Appendix E). If you state no preferences you will have to negotiate on the day and for some things it may be too late e.g. breastfeeding in theatre – your gown may be trapped by the screen unless you are clear you want skin-to-skin contact with your baby while still in surgery.

Caesareans can offer significant benefits in some situations so even if you really want to avoid one, recognise its potential in your birth plan and acknowledge it is a possible outcome of your birth. Realistic expectations increase the likelihood of you viewing your birth in a positive light should it change direction.[60]

> *"We'd left our childbirth classes believing very firmly that how our birth experience went was ultimately within our control. We were sorely misguided."*[59]
> Maureen Connolly, Birth Commentator et al

The following ideas do not constitute a full vaginal birth plan (see Other resources) rather concentrate solely on suggestions for trying to avoid a caesarean.

Avoid continual fetal heart monitoring

This technique provides immediate feedback on your baby's condition, essential if she is showing signs of distress. However it significantly restricts your movement and readings can be inaccurate. Natural fluctuations in your baby's heart rate occur as birth progresses. The experience of your midwife is important when interpreting these fluctuations. A *distress* diagnosis may simply be *natural fluctuation*. In some circumstances you may wish to request fetal blood sampling to determine whether the fluctuations actually reflect fetal distress. Fetal monitors should not be used as a matter of routine as continuous use has been connected with caesarean outcomes.[61] They should only be used when a need has been identified.[62] Though you will be monitored periodically if you have an epidural but this need not be continuous and is recommended only for 30 minutes as the anaesthetic gets established.[63]

Understand the impact of epidurals

Epidurals have been connected with a slight slowing of labour (2nd stage) for *some* women. [64] [65] This seems in part due to the use (in some hospitals) of continuous fetal heart monitoring rather than the epidural itself. Epidurals do not appear to increase the likelihood of instrumental intervention or caesarean[66] [67] [68] and can provide excellent pain relief, essential for some women. However, dosages that provide better pain relief also tend to reduce your mobility. If you want an epidural recognise that a lighter dosage, while enabling you to remain more mobile, may not achieve the level of pain relief you would prefer. Note – to avoid unnecessary pain your epidural need not be tailed off until "after completion of the third stage of labour and any necessary perineal repair" (UK NICE caesarean guideline[69]).

Avoid lying on your back

The weight of your baby can compress the vein that returns blood to your heart. This can make you faint and if compressed for a prolonged period can also disrupt your baby's oxygen supply causing distress. Lying in this position compresses your pelvis too, narrowing the space available for your baby to pass through and reducing contraction intensity while increasing their frequency.[70] Being upright adds gravity to those factors working with you in birth.

Plan a homebirth or labour at home for as long as possible

Early removal to hospital increases the likelihood of medical intervention.[71] Planned home births tend to have lower rates of intervention. Though remember planning a home birth is a preference not a guarantee.

Allow waters to break naturally

Avoiding artificial intervention reduces the risk of infection.

Avoid drugs to artificially speed up labour

A mother describing her first birth said "I was overdue and being monitored daily. The hospital decided to induce me and after three pessaries over two days, it was obvious nothing was happening so my waters were broken. Then I was put on a drip that they cranked up as things were still very slow and given an epidural. After two days of this he started to show signs of distress and was born by emergency caesarean." Anna (31)

Artificially stimulated contractions are typically stronger and some babies become distressed, leading to the need for a caesarean.

Avoid induction

Being induced increases the likelihood of other interventions such as continuous electronic fetal monitoring, epidurals and IVs. These practices restrict your movement, *may* slow your labour and *some* can, when coupled with increased fatigue from the strength and frequency of contractions, increase the likelihood of caesarean or instrumental intervention. If you have had a previous caesarean, induction is associated with higher uterine rupture rates.[72]

Induction

Induction contractions may not be any more painful than those of women who have gone into labour naturally. However, they may get stronger more quickly with less warning for each one, making it difficult to achieve effective pain relief with gas and air, increasing the likelihood of your requesting an epidural.

Eat and drink during labour

Some hospitals discourage this because it can cause difficulties for *some* women going on to need a general anaesthetic. Research clearly shows that for women with low risk pregnancies, light snacks, particularly fluids, are fine.[73] Isotonic drinks have been shown to provide valuable energy while not significantly increasing gastric volume.[74] Many practitioners now recognise that it is essential that you keep your strength up and remain hydrated and so encourage light snacks.

Set your own pace for pushing

Avoid pressure being exerted on the skin around the opening as your baby is crowning (baby's scalp is visible). The same applies to pressure on your abdomen (fundal pressure), though these practise are now relatively rare in any case.

Choose your care situation

Briefly, your options are home birth, hospital or midwife-led unit and you may choose to use the services of an independent midwife or doula. The type of support available in each of these varies so investigate each option:

- Think about the policies and the statistics of each

- Do your own research. Do not expect to be offered these options. You will need to investigate midwife-led units and doulas yourself. The Internet, your local health services and local community services should have information

- Talk to people who have taken the approach you are thinking of using

Home birth

A familiar environment may be more relaxing and feel safer for some women than hospital. Continuity of care can be good and your midwife sympathetic to your wish to avoid hospitalisation (particularly if you are employing your own midwife). UK NHS midwifery teams are obliged to support home births but may refer you to other midwives if they are not confident with your pregnancy circumstances.[75] It is important to consider how close your hospital is when choosing a home birth. If, during labour, you and/or your midwife decide that you now need hospital care you do not want to be 45 minutes from the nearest epidural or caesarean. It can mean the difference between life and death for you and/or your baby.

Vaginal birth in hospital

Some women prefer to give birth in hospital because their home does not feel appropriate (e.g. other siblings at home, lack of space or peace etc.). For others it is more to do with how confident they feel in their own abilities and their wish to be close to medical teams. Birth units offering *low tech, home-like* services are

Be open to change

Injury to you and your baby from forceps and ventouse can be significant (see Appendix C). If you find yourself facing this you may want to consider switching to a caesarean instead of opting for these interventions.

increasingly available in hospitals. These are next to or within the maternity ward but are individual rooms with space for birthing balls, softer lighting, warm colours, and some have a birthing pool included. When considering a hospital birth you may be able to choose from more than one in your area.

Midwife-led units

These tend to be small units offering a more *intimate* feel with a low tech approach to child birth. Individual rooms may contain a birth pool, shower and toilet and are likely to have extra touches like carpets and comfy chairs. There should be good continuity of care, but remember to consider, as for home births, the distance to the nearest hospital and, of course, the expense.

Hire independent support

The cost of independent support varies. So too can the type of cases they are able to support.

Midwives

Independent midwives can work with you for both home and hospital births (though once in hospital they can represent your preferences but can no longer direct your care). UK staffing levels vary across the country and despite a national recommendation of one midwife to every labouring woman[77] this cannot be guaranteed in many maternity units unless you take your own independent midwife with you. Independent midwives offer continuity of care and individualised preparation and aftercare.

> **Consider trained birth partners**
>
> "Women who received continuous labour support were more likely to give birth *spontaneously*, i.e. give birth with neither caesarean nor vacuum nor forceps. In addition, women were less likely to use pain medications, were more likely to be satisfied, and had slightly shorter labours." Dr Ellen Hodnett, Nursing Professor, University of Toronto [76] et al

Doula

These supporters provide assistance: before, during and after birth and studies have shown that having a doula present at your birth can reduce the likelihood of having a caesarean or instrumental delivery.[78] [79]

Turning your baby

If your baby is laying the *wrong way round*, i.e. she is sideways or bottom first, then a caesarean may be suggested. You can request waiting until labour begins (see Chapter 1) before agreeing, some babies do turn during labour. In addition there are a number of techniques you could try to encourage your baby to turn:

- **External Cephalic Version (ECV)** – This requires a trained practitioner. Pressure to your abdomen encourages your baby to turn. It is thought to work in about 50% of cases. ECV is not appropriate in all circumstances, for example if you have scars on your uterus from previous surgery, you are already bleeding or your baby is compromised in some way

- **Acupressure and acupuncture** – [More info.iii]

Other techniques may be suggested however bear in mind that they have not been clinically proven and *may* be risky without trained guidance:

- **Massage** – Ask your midwife to show you how to massage your belly in a clockwise direction applying gentle pressure at specific points. This should not be attempted without trained supervision as it can damage the placenta enough to require immediate induction or caesarean

- **Optimal fetal positioning** – This theory suggests your behaviour can influence your baby's position (see Other resources). [More info.iv]

Ask lots of questions

In addition to those issues described above, you may want to ask your practitioner about their definition of *active labour*, policies on fetal heart monitoring, fetal blood sampling etc. (see Appendix F).

If you are hoping to have a VBAC (see – this chapter), be aware that some hospitals actively discourage this and rates vary between hospitals so you may want to ask about this specifically.

Once in labour, continue to ask questions. If there is really no time for questions your situation is serious and probably does require immediate surgery. If there is still time for questions your situation is not yet critical. A good question to start with is "What if we do nothing?" or "Can we wait for another hour?"

Rest

Studies suggest that taking paid maternity leave in the 4 weeks leading up to your birth *may* reduce the need for a caesarean.[80] Certainly the more relaxed you feel, the more you will be able to concentrate on the preparation of your body and mind as well as your home.

---

iii Summary of studies www.breech.co.uk/thescience.php

iv www.homebirth.org.uk/ofp.htm

Investigate hypno-birthing

This technique appears to offer remarkable control over mind and body. You *may* be able to reduce pain, fear and anxiety whilst in labour, creating a calmer experience for yourself as well as a less stressed baby. Courses can be expensive and do not work for everyone. Fear of hospitals, needles, panic attacks and clinical depression can make your pregnancy and labour unpleasant. Hypnotherapy and psychotherapy can address such fears (see Other resources). Studies looking at the use of hypnosis in childbirth support this idea.[81] [82]

Stay healthy

Keep in good physical condition, eat well and take regular, appropriate exercise (see Chapter 5). You are more likely to have a caesarean if you are overweight (see Appendix C).

During labour keep your strength up by continuing to take fluids at the very least and eat light snacks.

Get hold of your previous medical notes

Obtain your notes from previous births, particularly if you are moving hospital. Providing information about a previous caesarean may help a VBAC request, particularly if the reason for it is not one that is likely to recur. If you have given birth vaginally before this increases your chances of success.[83] [84]

VBAC classes and support groups

There are some courses that concentrate on VBACs, though you may need to travel to access these. A search on the Internet will reveal what type of classes and support groups are in your area.

I am still being told a caesarean might be best

Clarify whether it is a *suggestion* or *necessity* and what it is about your specific case that leads to this conclusion. The term *complication* sounds frightening and can cover many things. Remember many grey areas exist and what is labelled a complication in one hospital is not necessarily the case in the birthing unit down the road. So ask lots of questions and include your birth partner in the discussion. If time permits get a second opinion. If you cannot come to terms with the possibility of a caesarean you may want to consider counselling to address the fears and concerns that are driving your thoughts.

Can I go against the advice of my practitioner?

As everyone's situation is different it is crucial you discuss your individual case with your practitioner until, time permitting, you are happy with the information you are being given. You may not find anyone willing to agree with your preference. This may be because you have been particularly unlucky or in medical terms you really are best advised to have a caesarean. If you have the time and resources you may want to broaden the number of people whose opinion you seek in order to make a more informed decision.

Make sure you understand your legal rights. These vary from country to country (see Chapter 3) and will have an impact upon whether or not you can insist upon a vaginal birth attempt.

Faced with the situation where all the feedback you are getting points to a caesarean there will come a time when you need to start planning for this. There are lots of things that you can do to make it feel a more special, personal and manageable experience (see Chapter 5). Afterwards you may benefit from support in getting over your birth. There are many ideas and resources available to you (see Chapter 6 & Other resources).

Vaginal Birth After Caesarean (VBAC)

There are whole books and websites dedicated to this aspect of birth (see Other resources), the following is just to get you started. Practitioner recommendations for a repeat caesarean can sound very compelling. You can refuse an intervention but be sure of your medical situation and your own reasons for doing so as well as the impact of your decision. Remember too that stating a desire to have a VBAC is a preference not a guaranteed outcome.

Can I have a VBAC?

It is not unusual to be told that if you have already had a caesarean, future babies should be born this way too. However a VBAC is increasingly available to women. Assuming you request this, figures currently suggest women meeting specific criteria are 75-80% likely to be successful.[85] If you have had more than one caesarean the VBAC success rate is fractionally lower

A mum's comment after an unplanned caesarean during a VBAC "Even though I really wanted a VBAC I am just relieved to be here. My daughter has a new brother, she still has a mother and my husband still has his wife." Vicki 38

but still above 70% and improves if you have also had a previous vaginal delivery,[86] [87] particularly if it was after the caesarean.[88] VBAC risks do not appear greater the more caesareans you have.[89]

Unfortunately some women are not aware that, in the UK at least, a vaginal birth is still a possibility after a caesarean – often believing the long held myth that *once a caesarean always a caesarean*. This coupled with strong recommendations by some practitioners further confuses the situation. That said recommendations from your practitioner should not be rejected without a clear understanding of the implications of attempting a VBAC in your case. In the US, lawyers and insurance companies can influence your options even more significantly and in 2010 9 out of 10 US women are routinely offered a caesarean.[90] It should be your specific situation not policies or practitioner preferences driving the decision but this is not always the case. In such circumstances arm yourself with as much information as you can so you stand the best chance of success.

If you meet the following criteria you are more likely to gain support for a VBAC:

- You have no medical condition currently requiring a caesarean

- Previous uterine incisions were horizontal and *not* vertical (the internal incision may be different from the external one)

- The reasons for your previous caesarean were specific to that pregnancy and unlikely to occur in the next

- You are not overweight

- You do not need to be induced

- You have not had a scar rupture previously

- You have not had more than 2 caesareans (though this factor is unclear and still a matter of opinion)

Despite agreement that it is safe for the majority of women, opinion on VBACs, particularly after 2 or more caesareans, is very divided and if your case is not straightforward (e.g. multiple births) you may have difficulty finding a practitioner prepared to support you. You may wish to seek a second opinion (see Chapter 3). [More info.[v]]

Before making a final decision ensure you understand the risks and benefits of both VBAC and repeat caesarean then check out the policies at your place of birth. It may be, for example, the hospital sets limits on the duration of first and second stages of labour. As long as your labour is progressing well and you and your baby are not showing signs of distress there is no reason why you should be restricted to arbitrary timescales.[91] [More info.[vi]]

> *A mum's experience of a VBAC*
> *"Giving birth to C was the most amazing experience of my life. Seeing her little face and watching her turn pink in my arms is something I shall remember vividly forever."*
> *Caroline 29*

---

[v] www.rcog.org.uk search for Birth After Previous Caesarean – Green top 45

[vi] Churchill H, Savage W 'Vaginal Birth After Caesarean' 2008 Middlesex University Press ISBN-13: 978-1904750215

What are the benefits of a VBAC?

- Increased chance of vaginal birth in future pregnancies
- Avoidance of surgery risks (see Appendix C)
- Labour ideally begins naturally
- Possible decrease in the likelihood of respiratory problems for your baby (see Appendix C)
- Potentially shorter stay in hospital
- Possibility of shorter recovery period
- Sense of achievement and fulfilment

What are the benefits of a planned repeat caesarean?

- "Virtually no risk of scar rupture" (Royal College of Obstetricians & Gynaecologists[92])
- Lower risk of blood transfusion[93] and fetal death or brain damage[94]
- Previous experience of the procedure means you may face it and the recovery more calmly and knowledgably
- *Damage* is confined to the same area as before

What are the risks associated with a VBAC?

Some situations appear to reduce the likelihood of success, but research is inconclusive in the areas of maternal weight, induction and larger babies. [More info.[vii]]

In addition to those risks associated with any vaginal birth (see Appendix C) there are a number of additional risks specific to VBACs:

- **Failed vaginal attempt** – Unplanned caesareans occur in 1 in 4 attempted VBACs[96] and you are twice as likely to experience health problems including bladder and bowel laceration in such situations[97]

> **Implications of failed vaginal birth attempts**
>
> "63.6 percent of major complications and 28.4 percent of minor complications occurred in women who required caesarean section after an unsuccessful trial of labour." Dr Michael J. McMahon, University of North Carolina School of Medicine[95] et al

vii Churchill H, Savage W 'Vaginal Birth After Caesarean' 2008 Middlesex University Press ISBN-13: 978-1904750215

- **Negative emotional response** – Converting to an unplanned caesarean during a VBAC can be very emotionally distressing for *some* women, particularly so for those who really wanted to avoid another caesarean. Recognising that a caesarean is a possible outcome of any birth and planning with this in mind can reduce the emotional trauma experienced by *some* women, (see Chapter 5)

- **Scar rupture** – The incidence of scar rupture is very low, less than 22-74 in 10,000.[98] For horizontal scars the risk is so low that alone this should not be used as a reason against a VBAC (see Appendix C). The risk is increased if you need to be induced.[99] However if a rupture is identified bleeding can be heavy and life-threatening and an emergency caesarean will be necessary

- **Blood transfusions** – The risk is higher (17 in 1,000) than for a planned caesarean (10 in 1,000) [100])

> *A mum describing her plans following a traumatic emergency caesarean said of next time "I really wanted a VBAC however the consultant I saw at 28 weeks did not seem impressed with this but agreed to me trying, only allowing me 10-12 hours labour time. My waters broke naturally but I did not progress and once again ended up with a caesarean. Knowing what to expect I was calmer and my milk came in very quickly this time. I put this down to being more relaxed second time round." Anne (32)*

- **Endometritis** – The risk is higher (28 in 1,000) than for a planned caesarean (18 in 1,000) [101]

- **Medical conditions** – There is a higher risk of an unplanned caesarean due to the increased chance of complications such as placenta praevia and placenta accreta after previous caesareans (see Appendix C). You may wish to request additional scans to check. If you have either condition there is little chance of a VBAC

- **Maternal death** – Extremely rare[102 103] (see Appendix C)

- **Death of baby** – Extremely rare but higher than the risk associated with planned repeat caesareans (see Appendix C)

What are the risks associated with a planned repeat caesarean?

The risks associated with planned repeat caesareans are the same as for any planned caesarean (see Appendix C) though the likelihood of developing a condition associated with the placenta leading to complications increases the more caesareans you have. In addition there are the following risks:

- The procedure may be slightly longer due to scar tissue from previous surgery
- There is an increased likelihood of caesareans for future births

CHAPTER FIVE

How can I make the most of my caesarean?

Planning for the arrival of your baby can be very exciting. In addition to dreaming about the baby growing inside you, you may be thinking about cots versus bed-sharing, home versus hospital birthing options, breast versus bottle feeding etc. There are many books and websites discussing all of these. However in many cases these will concentrate almost exclusively on vaginal birth.

A caesarean can place additional demands upon both you and your support network. There are key things to learn and prepare for with this mode of birth. Whether you are planning one or not, appropriate antenatal preparation can help you *feel* more in control, making for a more positive experience and recovery[104] Preparing for the period beyond your birth can remove some of the worry about how you will manage. Ultimately, planning for the possibility of a caesarean means, should you have one, all those parts of your birth for which you can express a preference can be discussed and agreed in advance.

What is a birth plan?

A birth plan is a document created by you to describe your birth preferences. Working your way through one is the easiest way to ensure you have thought about your options and are well prepared. Realistic preparation is linked with lower rates of emotional birth trauma.[105] However, you should *not* assume that preparing a birth plan will guarantee exactly the birth you want.

"The first time round was a nightmare. I ended up with a caesarean after 22 hours of labour. I couldn't face going through that again so I had an elective caesarean this time...I was still worried beforehand but in comparison to last time I knew what to expect and I was much more relaxed. I cuddled him in theatre, amazing." Cheryl (28)

Every birth is different so you can never truly predict what will happen or how you will feel on the day. With this in mind do not include anything that closes down options e.g. "I do not want an epidural under any circumstances". A protracted, difficult birth can make even the most pro-natural birth proponent call for the anaesthetist.

How to write a birth plan

Headings

Make it easy for people to find the relevant section in a hurry. If you are using a template make sure it includes all the issues important to you. Keep it short – a bullet list is easier to read than paragraphs.

Templates

Try using the hospital template if one is available. Your practitioner will be familiar with the format making it easier to refer to.

Research

Talk to friends who have already been through birth. Find out what they found important, what worked and what did not. Some things will strike a chord with you, some things will not. Talk to your practitioners too and make sure you understand what they consider *standard practice* at your hospital. This may suggest things you might prefer to be done slightly differently. It may be particularly useful to talk to those mothers who have given birth at the same hospital.

> **Manage your expectations**
>
> "Recognising that a caesarean is a possibility in any pregnancy and understanding the possible reasons for it may make women feel less traumatised emotionally if their delivery suddenly becomes a surgical event, even if the decision for surgery is made very rapidly, to save a life or lives." Dr Michele Moore, Physician in preventative care and women's health[106] et al

Get agreement

Involve your birth partner – they should be familiar with the plan (and agree with it). Discuss it with your practitioners too – it may be that some preferences are not possible in your situation. If you have not gained agreement in advance it may not be possible to accommodate them once in labour/surgery, particularly if they are unusual. Your practitioners may be able to suggest alternatives. Even those aspects of birth you are hoping to avoid could have alternatives agreed e.g. if a ventouse is suggested during a vaginal birth you may agree that there should be no episiotomy. Where situations change quickly you may not have time or feel able to work through the issues before deciding on a course of action. In preparing a plan you will have thought through many things already. While birth plans

> **Plan for every eventuality**
>
> Even if you are hoping to avoid a caesarean, plan for its possibility. "The women most prone to post caesarean depression are those who during pregnancy were most determined not to have one." Dr Kathryn Cox, Obstetrics & gynaecology[107] et al

are increasingly popular and accepted there are still practitioners who are not particularly interested in them. Where this is the case you may feel strongly enough to request a different practitioner.

Timing

A birth plan should be written and agreed well in advance of your due date. *Do not* just hand it over on the day.

Wording

Take care with your wording - aggressive language and sweeping statements about things you will not tolerate may antagonise.

Sign off

When everything is agreed ask your practitioners to sign it. Make sure those signing are actually in a position to do so. Give them a copy and keep copies for yourself with your hospital bag. Have spares to hand out to additional staff as necessary.

What can I include in a caesarean birth plan?

The following list is not in any particular order. Only include those preferences that really strike a chord with you otherwise the plan will become very unwieldy. The following ideas are specifically for caesareans but you will find lots of vaginal birth plans on the internet (see Other resources).

A general statement

Unless you have agreed to a planned caesarean (without labour) you may want to state preferences about the way in which your vaginal birth can move to a caesarean should it become necessary. For example, you may wish to indicate that you are not averse to a caesarean and would prefer this to forceps and ventouse intervention.

Natural caesarean

This procedure offers the potential of a slower, calmer delivery and gives you the ability to personalise aspects of your birth (see Chapter 1). This type of delivery is only possible in straightforward, planned caesareans and is not offered as a matter of routine, so if you are interested, discuss it well in advance.

Delivery date

Agree to a date *no earlier* than week 39 unless medical reasons indicate your baby needs to be delivered earlier (see Appendix B & Appendix C).

To labour or not to labour

Do you want to go into labour before the caesarean or would you rather avoid it? There are implications for both (see Chapter 1 & Appendix C). If you want to labour, clarify how long for. Remember that staff and theatre availability will mean that you will need to be flexible on the day.

People present

State if you want to have a birth partner present. If you wish to have more than one (e.g. a doula or independent midwife) agree this specifically. Some hospitals allow only one person in theatre with you if space is limited. If you require a general anaesthetic, your birth partner will be asked to leave theatre although your doula or independent midwife *may* be allowed to stay. If you are in a teaching hospital you may find students will be observing unless you state a preference against this. Think about whether you really want them excluded. They need to learn and they could photograph the birth for you.

Screen placement

The screen is there to prevent accidental contamination of the sterile operating area and to obscure your view of surgery. It can sometimes be lowered at the point of delivery so you can see your baby being lifted out. If you are hoping to hold/feed her in theatre ask that the screen be positioned as low as possible. It is unlikely to be possible to insert a screen once surgery has begun so be certain before asking for no screen at all.

Upper body mobility

Ensure your gown opens at the front and that it is not trapped underneath the screen if you are hoping to breastfeed or hold your baby skin-to-skin. Check your arms are not going to be restricted (other than the IV drip) and that monitors are attached to your back rather than your chest.

Anaesthesia

Only state a preference following detailed discussion with your anaesthetist. They may have preferences in which they are more skilled or there may be a hospital policy directing the type of anaesthetic. It is important you understand the implications of each type, as their impact upon you can be very different. A general anaesthetic is not standard practice carrying higher risks (see Appendix C). You will need very good reasons for requesting a general if this is your preference.

Catheter

Clarify that the catheter is inserted *after* the epidural takes effect – it can be uncomfortable otherwise.

Prophylactic antibiotics

In many hospitals these are administered as a matter of routine and have been proven effective in reducing the incidence of postoperative infection.[108] [109] If you are concerned about the impact of antibiotics on your baby these can be administered *after* the umbilical cord has been cut or you can reject them altogether. However, understand that infection can be distressing and uncomfortable until antibiotic treatment can take effect and this may have an impact upon how well you feel and a knock on affect on your ability to breastfeed.

The cord

Who is going to cut it – you, your birth partner or the surgeon? This must be agreed in advance so they can easily ensure the surgical site remains sterile. When would you prefer it to be cut? This may be determined by the circumstances of your caesarean (speed may be important), hospital policy, the preference of your surgeon or you may be able to request a 2 minute delay. Controlled cord traction is standard practice in the UK as it reduces the risk of endometritis.[112] You may want to check hospital policy on this.

Delayed cord cutting

Delaying for 2 minutes[110] [111] is thought to enable valuable oxygen and nutrients (e.g. iron) to continue to reach your baby until breathing has been properly established, also reducing the risk of anaemia. This is an ongoing debate but if you have a particular view, state your preference in advance as it can be quite difficult to gain agreement for this.

Incision and stitches

Most hospitals use the *bikini* cut, a horizontal cut in your bikini line – unless your condition dictates a vertical incision (see Appendix C). Closure techniques vary so check your hospital's policy. If dissolvable stitches are not being used find out why. The alternatives are staples, clips or non-disposable stitches, all of which will need to be removed after a few days, which some women find uncomfortable. Cosmetically there appears to be little[113] to "no difference in both subjective and objective scar rating...at either 2 months or 6 months" (Dr Antonella Cromi, University of Insurbia, Italy[114]).

Baby's arrival

At the moment of birth, you may wish to ask for quiet and dimmed lights. This is *may* be possible, though unlikely in emergencies. It is common practice to have music playing in theatre so supply your own CD if you have particular preferences.

Who holds your baby?

You can ask for your baby to be passed to you before she is cleaned and checked, though medical concerns may mean this is not advisable. In most cases your baby will remain in the same room. If she needs to be taken elsewhere agree with your birth partner in advance whether you want them to stay with you or go with your baby. One advantage of a doula is she can stay with you while your birth partner goes with your baby or vice versa. You may wish to wash and dress your baby yourself once back on the ward – state this if so.

Your placenta

It is not standard practice to view your placenta so specify this if you want to, particularly if you want to take it away with you.

Who discovers the sex of your baby?

You can choose to discover the sex of your baby yourself or be told by your surgeon.

Do you want a visual record of your birth?

Photographs need to be agreed in advance. Cameras are generally permissible but video cameras may be less so. Agree who is going to take the photos, your birth partner may prefer to be concentrating on the actual birth and it may be a good idea to turn the flash off to avoid making people jump. In the case of a general anaesthetic you may benefit later from having photos of your birth as you will not have any awareness of it at the time.

Special care unit

If you know that your baby will go to SCU after birth you may want to visit in advance so you can imagine her there before you are able to visit her. You may also want to have a photo taken of her so you have something with you on the ward. Looking at an image of your baby can help *letdown* when you are expressing breast milk.

> *A mum describing an unplanned caesarean with a general said "I woke up sometime later and there he was. None of it is clear to me. I feel incredibly sad that I have no memory of his birth. What can I tell him - nothing."* Sarah (37)

Who wakes you

If you are having a general anaesthetic your anaesthetist will remain with you until you wake but you may wish to request your birth partner waits in recovery with you too and perhaps is the one to bring your baby to you. You will be a little groggy when you wake so if you use a different name to the one on your records say so to avoid confusion as you wake.

Breastfeeding

Make your position on breastfeeding clear whatever your opinion. Breastfeeding is actively encouraged in most places so pain relief should be compatible, but check. If you want to avoid formula make this clear too. Well-meaning midwives may give your baby formula if you are asleep or still unconscious after a general anaesthetic or particularly difficult birth. You can express milk during your time in hospital to be used if you are sleeping. Whichever your preference it is worth reminding staff as each shift changes.

What to wear

While hospital gowns are rather like tents they are functional and serviceable. Save your own lying-in clothes for the ward.

Where does my baby sleep?

In most hospitals your baby is with you on the ward. Unless one of you requires a special care unit, a bassinette can be placed by your bed so your baby can remain with you at all times. Some hospitals have three sided cots that can be clipped onto your bed making it much easier for you to move your baby towards you, if you want one you will need to request it. You may also wish to discuss options for keeping your baby in bed with you.

Where do I sleep?

You may want to request a private room for most of your stay in hospital. Most places will not allow you to use it in the first 24 hours, as they need to keep a very close eye on you and prefer to do this on the ward. The number of rooms is often limited and unlikely to be free of charge. Bear in mind that out of sight you will have to ring and wait for assistance as you are less likely to catch a nurse or midwife as they pass.

How can I prepare for a caesarean birth?

Knowing you are having a caesarean or simply acknowledging the possibility means you can prepare yourself and your home accordingly. Other forms of medical intervention can create similar challenges to those you might experience with a caesarean birth and you may benefit from some of these ideas after a vaginal birth too.

> *"I made a decision before my second birth [after a previous emergency caesarean] that I had to prepare better. I did not bond with D and I think it's because of the trauma. I did not want it to be like that with G too." Hannah (28)*

Things to learn before your birth

Learn about caesareans

Knowing even the basics can reduce anxiety. Unplanned caesareans can happen when you are least able to take in information and feel least in control of your body or environment. In these circumstances the less information that is completely new the better. For example: knowing beforehand the difference between *failure to progress* and your baby *being in distress* means you can talk knowledgeably about your options while continuing to labour (or not) (see Appendix B). Given this make sure you understand:

- The different types of caesarean and how the experience can vary (see Chapter 1)

- What the benefits and risks of a caesarean are (see Appendix C)

- The reasons why a caesarean may be recommended (see Appendix B)

- What your rights are (see Chapter 3)

- The terminology (see Chapter 1)

- What will happen and where you can express a preference (see Chapter 5 & Appendix A)

- What recovery may be like (see Chapter 6)

Why the caesarean is necessary

With a planned caesarean make sure you understand the reasons for the recommendation and whether it is a matter of opinion (see Appendix B). For example: a baby lying breech does not automatically require a caesarean. Allow yourself time, if need be, to grieve the vaginal birth you will not have, and then plan a positive birth experience.

Flexibility

Everyone develops a view of the way they want to give birth. Recognising this can only ever be a preference is an important factor in preparing. Your views can affect your behaviour during labour[115] and will play an important part in how you feel as you recover. I cannot stress enough the importance of being open to change and acknowledging that birth is a bit of a lottery. Research suggests that having realistic expectations means you are less likely to experience *extreme* forms of disappointment post operatively[116] (as can being involved in the decision-making process and your interpretation of your control). [117] [118] [119]

You have a 1 in 4 (UK) [120] or 1 in 3 (USA)[121] chance of having a caesarean. Try to view it as the life-saving procedure it often is. With a vaginal birth make plans but maintain an element of flexibility so if your circumstances change you have taken account of caesarean birth and have preferences agreed.

Understand interventions

Research suggests that antenatally some women are increasingly viewing intervention (particularly epidurals) more positively.[123] Intervention of one sort or another occurs in over 50% of UK births.[124] So while it is good to be open-minded, it is important to understand the implications of interventions before agreeing or asking for them, particularly if you are hoping for a vaginal birth. Interventions carry additional risks and *some* have been specifically connected with an increased likelihood of needing a caesarean (see Appendix C).

> **Manage your expectations**
>
> "Childbirth outcomes are a function of antenatal attitudes and feelings as well as of the events of labour." Josephine Green, Deputy Director at Mother & Infant Research Unit, University of Leeds[122] et al. In other words your preconceptions can play a significant part in how you manage, interpret and cope with your birth.

Involve your birth partner

Involve them as much as you both feel comfortable with. In many cases the birth partner is also the future parent so will likely have lots of questions and concerns about the birth and life afterwards too. If tackled openly and honestly this shared time can help reinforce your relationship and prepare you both for the forthcoming

> *A Mum commenting on her antenatal class said "It [a caesarean] was painted as a last resort. We weren't even really told it was a possibility, though we had been told about the instruments. I believed everything was going to be a nice normal birth." Janice (31)*

upheaval. They may wish to attend classes and antenatal appointments with you. Listen to their hopes and fears and give them the opportunity to voice these without dismissing them as *trivial by comparison.*

What will happen afterwards

Knowing the typical issues you may face while recovering from a caesarean can greatly reduce the worry that may otherwise arise when your body behaves differently to expected. Understand the sensations, why you are having them (or not), and how to manage your daily life (see Chapter 6). Understandably, some mothers experiencing unplanned caesareans blame the caesarean for the difficulties and sensations. This is not necessarily fair or realistic – some things will be the same whichever way you give birth. Blaming the caesarean can significantly affect your emotional recovery and may affect bonding, breastfeeding etc. Taking care of yourself properly during your recovery and having realistic expectations about your abilities can reduce physical distress and resentment (see Chapter 6).

Antenatal classes

These typically cover the options and complexities of vaginal birth and recovery. They may cover caesareans to the same degree but this is unusual. Despite research emphasising the importance and significance of realistic expectations,[125] [126] it is likely you will be given only basic information about caesareans. In order to develop a more balanced view

A mum talking about an antenatal class for her first birth said "The [antenatal] teacher crowded all the class around one of us and said how do you feel? To which she replied 'intimidated'. That was the sum total of what we were told about caesareans." Isabel (36)

you will need to read around the subject, using books like this and others (see Other resources). That said, antenatal classes will teach breathing and relaxation techniques which can be very useful, particularly when you are in hospital waiting for your caesarean. Attending classes run by your hospital and local midwifery teams will also give you a better idea of the attitudes and personal opinions of your potential carers. Private classes may be more tailored to your specific needs and perspectives.

Make new friends

Having even a couple of friends at a similar stage of pregnancy gives you someone to share ideas and concerns with. Most places run antenatal classes and these are a good way to meet up.

Breastfeeding positions

After a caesarean you are likely to feel sore across your abdomen. Alternatives to traditional feeding positions may suit you better. Try these out beforehand so you feel more competent when it's time to use them (see Chapter 6).

"Those 24 or so hours of birth are significant but perhaps not nearly as significant as the 18 years of childcare that follow. The birth is only the beginning of a whole new chapter in your life..." Christa Greenacre, (NCT teacher – retired)

Self-hypnosis

Learning this technique can be useful before, during and after birth. Self-hypnosis can be used to help you remain or regain a state of calm. Whether you are labouring or waiting for a planned caesarean, staying calm will be very important to your state of mind as you go forward (see Other resources).

Things to do before going to hospital

Deal with fear

It is natural to be apprehensive about birth. You have hopes and dreams but these are coloured by the stories and anecdotes both real and make believe that you have encountered through friends and the media. If your antenatal class focused on drug-free birth you may be quite fearful about caesareans, but viewing a caesarean as a failure or a massive loss of control is not helpful. Many of the underlying feelings and worries are the same as those experienced before a vaginal birth: Will I cope? Will my baby be ok? Will it hurt?

Seek support if you feel your fear is getting in the way of enjoying your pregnancy. Counselling can tackle the fears and their underlying causes, alleviating some of the problems. If you have had a previous traumatic birth or suffered physical/sexual abuse, this is particularly important. Studies show that birth experience can be a healing experience for some women but the pain and perceived humiliation can also *re-traumatise*

> *A mum talking about her first birth said "Having heard so many friends' terrible birth stories I started to question my body's abilities. I wanted a small family and after lots of reading came to the conclusion that for me the only way to do it was by planning a caesarean." Jenny (34)*

others (see Appendix B & Appendix D). Perhaps consider hypnotherapy to help face birth more calmly. In accessing accurate and realistic antenatal information many women can *feel* more in control of their decision-making before and during labour. This *feeling* of control is very important, helping some women to develop a positive interpretation of their birth even if it has not gone to plan.[127]

Clear perspective

The focus of childbirth ought to be the safe delivery of your baby, but it is easy to dwell instead on the experience itself e.g. breathing and massage, a general feeling of calm in a cosy room with soft lighting, far from drugs and

> *"My mother had three very easy home births and I expected to follow suit." Anna (31)*

doctors. While some births do happen in circumstances like these, many do not. In the grand scheme of things the job you make of raising your baby is far more important than the way you gave birth to her, yet all too often women focus almost exclusively on the birth itself forgetting there are things to learn about the days and weeks that will follow. In any case there is a very real possibility you will change your approach as your birth progresses, or your birth could take a u-turn, needing induction, instruments etc. There is no shame in this. In the past women died. Now this is extremely rare, thanks in the main to the successes of modern interventions including caesareans.

Talk to your practitioners

Get a variety of perspectives. This way you can ensure that you have a more rounded view of what is ahead. Talk to an anaesthetist about your pain relief options, perhaps talk to more than one midwife. Make sure you understand your range of options.

Think about maternity leave

Have a rough idea of what may happen in the next few months. Worrying about work while on maternity leave is going to add unnecessary stress. Before your birth, if possible, iron out issues of maternity cover, additional childcare for siblings and childcare for your new baby if you are returning to work within 6 months etc.

Who is there on the day

Agree with your birth partner how they want to be involved in the birth (see Chapter 7). In addition to your birth partner you may want to consider a doula. Doulas can support you during birth and their familiarity can be very calming. They are not responsible for your medical care but are there to support you in your choices and actively assist you throughout. Beforehand they can help find ways to manage your birth and achieve those preferences you have specified. During a caesarean they may provide a running commentary about what is going on around you, stay with you while your baby is taken for checks or take pictures for you, provide massage to help you relax etc. Their role is to support you and your birth partner through the birth. Postnatally she may help you with breastfeeding and getting used to caring for your baby. [More info.[viii]]

> ### Understand your options
>
> Consultant involvement in pregnancies that are progressing normally is often limited. "This has meant that many women meet an obstetrician for the first time in the second stage of labour, with little understanding of the potential choices available for management." Deirdre J Murphy, Professor Obstetrics and Gynaecology, University of Dundee[128] et al. Knowing your options will help you have a rational informed discussion with your consultant.

Extra help at home

Once back at home you will be rather slow moving around and should not be lifting anything heavier than your baby. You should not be pushing a vacuum cleaner or catering for visitors. You may want to involve family and friends during the first weeks to ensure you do not put undue strain on

---

[viii] www.doula.org.uk

your abdomen as this will hamper your recovery. When asking people to help make sure they understand they are not coming just to cuddle your baby but to do the things that you cannot. They are there to help, not to make more work for you or create additional stress, so choose helpers with care. Arrange who helps/visits when and for how long, *before* you give birth to avoid confusion and pressure. In addition to help with meal times, general household tasks, food shopping etc. you will need to plan for sibling care. You will not be able to drive for several weeks so you will need to plan school pickups and trips to swimming lessons etc.

Stay healthy

Continue with moderate exercise as long as you feel able. Check your exercise plans with professionals to ensure you are not putting undue stress on yourself or your unborn baby. Eat healthily and get lots of sleep.

Prepare your nest

Your mobility will be impaired for a few days once back at home, so prepare a space to *nest*. In this area make sure you have everything you think you might need. You are going to spend a lot of time sitting feeding or cat napping so make it as comfortable and useful as possible. The sort of things you might include are: books, tissues, breast pads and breast cream, telephone, TV remotes, snugly blanket (for you), spare pillow (for you and for when feeding), snacks and jug of water/cup etc. These should all be within arm's length of the sofa as getting up and down frequently can quickly wear you out.

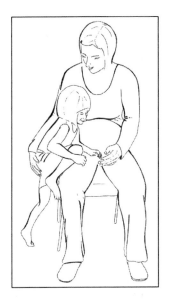

Figure 1 - Help them climb

Preparing toddlers

They are not going to understand that you are slower on your feet. Plan stationary activities – have a stock of things ready e.g. colouring books, crafts, story books, board games, modelling clay. Perhaps arrange extra, unaccompanied play dates for them, getting them used to a friend's house before you have your baby. As your bump gets bigger it is going to become more difficult to pick them up so make changes accordingly before your baby arrives e.g. sitting on the rug for a cuddle or helping them enjoy scrambling onto your lap rather than being lifted (see Figure 1). Make things funny rather than emphasising the necessity of them. Age appropriate books can get them used to the idea that a new baby will be arriving sometime soon (see Other resources).

Prepare older children

Explain to them that you are going to be a bit sore after their sister arrives and you are not going to be able to run around for a while (not that you are likely to have been doing this in the last month or so in any case). Talk in general terms about some of the practical changes that will happen, who will be taking them to school/swimming etc. Try to achieve a balance with them being *helpers* and still your children that need to *be children.*

Baby care

Minimise trips around the house by collecting together the things you need to keep your baby clean and warm. She is going to need complete changes (i.e. not just her nappy) several times, day and night. Consider setting up a couple of changing areas around the house, at least until you are more mobile. Have one in the room you are going to spend most of your time in and another where she will sleep. Perhaps include: nappies/diapers, wipes, bottom cream, changing mat, small towel, nappy bags and several changes of clothes replaced each day. Make sure changing areas are waist height to avoid unnecessary bending over as this can place additional strain on your abdominal muscles and incision as they heal.

> **Preparing friends and family**
>
> If you have planned a caesarean you may want to tell people when it is. If you do, make sure they understand that as a planned caesarean you will go in at a certain time, but surgery will be dependent upon theatre availability. The all important phone call may be much later than they expect.

Where to sleep

If you decide she is not going to sleep in your bed then you will need to have cleared space for a cot or moses basket. It is worth having this next to your bed so you can reach her without getting up if breastfeeding at night. Cots with collapsible sides are great – you can simply slide her towards you when she needs a feed. Bottle feeding will require more involvement from your partner in the beginning as you may feel less stable going up and down stairs carrying a baby and bottles.

Getting about

You will need a car seat, one with approved safety ratings, to bring your baby home. Fit it in advance. The last thing you want is to stand on the hospital steps (you will not be in a position to fiddle with it yourself) while someone else struggles and bounces your sleeping baby around in an increasingly desperate attempt to clip things in place. You may feel like taking short walks within days of being at home and while it might be your intention to carry your baby in a papoose/sling eventually, this might feel too much for the first day or so, so have your pram ready.

Talk to friends

Friends and family are a great source of ideas and information. You will of course get to hear their birth stories again but in between you will hear little nuggets of information that may really help you prepare.

Visit the hospital

This is important whichever way you plan to give birth. You may not have been inside a hospital in a long time and so only have the chaos of TV dramas in mind. Most hospitals offer trips around their maternity facilities. If you are hoping to birth at home then a hospital is not going to feel warm and cosy by comparison but by visiting, it at least becomes familiar. If you can, talk to women who have recently given birth there. You will be on the postnatal ward for several days and they will know how things work e.g. breakfast is often very early on hospital wards (7am) and knowing this you may choose to take breakfast snacks with you instead in case, by some miracle, you are still asleep at 7am.

Valuables

Leave them at home. Wedding rings will be taped down during surgery if necessary but all other jewellery will need to be removed and there is nowhere for you to safely store such things.

Hygiene

You may be shaved prior to surgery. You may want to do this yourself at home if you would prefer to avoid a cheap disposable razor in a nearby loo by the nearest nurse. You need only shave to the top of your bikini line and scissors rather than a razor may help avoid nicks – which can cause infection. You may want to shave or wax your legs and cut your toenails before you go in to hospital, assuming you can still reach them or even care. It is going to be a week or more before you feel able to stretch to that part of your body. There is no point having a pedicure or manicure though as nail polish is often removed before surgery.

Food

In the 48 hours leading up to a planned caesarean you may want to consider only eating easily digestible foods. This reduces the likelihood of gas building up in your digestive system. Gas can become worse after a caesarean and for some women can actually be more painful than the surgical recovery if it cannot be dislodged. Medication can alleviate this but it is better if it can be prevented in the first place.

What to take into hospital with you

In no particular order, things to pack for you:

- Your birth plan

- Several pairs of pyjamas or nightdresses (all loose round the waist and easy access at the front for feeding)

- Slippers and thick socks

- Dressing gown (and a cardigan for in bed)

- Loads of large knickers/panties – real *belly warmers* so the elastic comes above your belly button, you do not want anything rubbing the incision area

- Maternity pads (at least 1 pack) these are extra long to accommodate the fact that you will be lying down for longer and bleeding more than during a regular period

- Breast pads and nipple cream to help avoid cracked nipples

- 1 nursing bra (no more at this stage as you cannot predict your size and shape until you really start feeding)

- Hand mirror (you may not make it to the bathroom the first day)

- Face wipes or flannel (same reason)

- Toiletries are not provided so take your usual stash (assuming they are not too perfumed, you do not want to confuse your baby when you next pick her up – smell is a big thing for her until she can see properly). Breastfeeding can make your skin feel dry quickly so perhaps include lip balm and skin cream (unscented)

- A small pillow (or folded towel) to protect the incision from kicking feet when feeding (it is also good to hold over your incision when you cough or laugh)

- Hospital pillows may not be that great so you may want to bring one. An extra pillow can also help position you better when breastfeeding

- Headphones with a music player. Postnatal wards can be noisy and it can be frustrating listening to another baby cry when yours is sleeping. Other people's visitors are not always considerate and you can drown out conversation and take a doze with your headphones on

- Peppermint tea and fruit. As you are likely to be constipated and have trapped gas, these can help get your system moving more quickly

- Snacks. It is usual to be *nil by mouth* prior to a planned caesarean. Once back on the ward you may not coincide with a mealtime for hours. This and breastfeeding can make you hungry so ask visitors to keep your supplies stocked up. Include fruit and *non-fizzy* drinks in the snack box

- Things to do when your visitors are gone or your baby is asleep. Ideally you will be napping but magazines and books can fill what can sometimes be quite long periods on your own. These also come in handy if your planned caesarean is delayed for several hours

- Going home clothes, including your feeding bra. Avoid dresses unless they are specifically designed for breastfeeding and remember you will still be larger than pre-pregnancy (sizing about 6-7 months pregnant), so do not expect to fit into anything fancy (unless you buy it in a larger size). Do not expect to get into pre-pregnancy shoes either unless you have been cramming your feet into them during pregnancy. High heels are definitely out after a caesarean – they require far too much effort from your stomach muscles at this stage

- Makeup may seem like a really low priority and it probably is, but remember everyone will be wanting to take pictures of you and your baby when they visit. A little effort may make you feel less horrified when you look back at the photos later

- Coins for the phone (though mobiles are allowed in some hospital wards – do use them considerately)

- List of people you want to contact with your news

Before listing the things to pack for your baby, I would say do not go mad buying lots of everything. You do not know what size she is really going to be. Some newborn clothing is not going to fit a baby of 9lbs or more:

- Nappies/diapers (above size rule applies)

- Baby clothes (sleep suits and wrap over vests – easier than over the head ones, above size-rule applies)

- A smelly blanket. It may sound strange, but in some situations it is not always possible for you to have skin-to-skin time with your baby straight after birth. So wrapping her in a small blanket that smells of you will help reassure her. She will need covering in a warm blanket while laying skin-to-skin with you in theatre so it will be useful in any case

- Muslins (several as these may get covered in baby vomit very quickly)

- Cotton wool (rather than wipes for newborn nappy changing)

- Scratch mitts (some babies nails can be quite long at birth)
- Small blanket and hat for travelling home

What if I still do not feel ready?

You are likely to feel some anxiety leading up to your birth whether you are facing a planned caesarean or a vaginal birth. It may be the prospect of impending motherhood, worry about the birth, or having your home ready in time. Whichever it is, going through the checklists will at least ensure you have prepared the essentials. Counselling or hypnosis *may* help you deal with some anxiety but really it comes down to trusting yourself and those around you and being as positive as you can.

Remember – a caesarean is *not* a failure, it is simply another route to the safe delivery of your baby. This can be difficult to get your head round if you really want to birth vaginally but a critical one if you want to reduce the likelihood of emotional difficulties after your birth. *Own* your caesarean and try to see it as your route to motherhood.

> *"When everything changed so suddenly and she was born at 37 weeks I found that all the things I had bought were way too big. She grew into them of course but P had to do a mad dash to the shops for really small things in the mean time."*
> *Charlotte (24)*

CHAPTER SIX

How can I improve my recovery?

Your recovery from a caesarean is dependent upon a number of factors:

- The circumstances in which you had a caesarean
- How the caesarean progressed
- How much you knew about caesareans before experiencing one
- How much you were able to influence the experience
- Your preconceptions of birth and view of medical intervention
- How much help you had in the weeks afterwards

You can actually control several of these and this perception of control can go a long way in helping you cope with the caesarean and your physical and emotional recovery.

Your physical recovery

Many of the issues discussed here can be a *feature* of *any* pregnancy and birth. Where something is a result of a particular mode of birth this is indicated. It can really help first-time mothers who have an unplanned caesarean to know that some of the strange sensations are associated with *any* birth and are not the fault of the caesarean. This knowledge can reduce the resentment/disappointment that is sometimes associated with an unplanned caesarean.

Sensations after the birth

The following list shows the spectrum of sensations. Every birth is different just as every woman is and you may not experience these to the same degree described. Your experience will be dependent upon factors specific to you: birth circumstances, previous level of fitness, pain threshold, care taken during recovery, support afterwards, timeliness of pain medication etc.

The following list applies to vaginal birth recovery just as much as caesareans (with the sole exception of the incision issues). After a vaginal birth there will be pain and discomfort, bleeding and itching, just in different areas (see Appendix C).

Pain

Within the first few hours this may be anything from severe discomfort/pain and feeling unable to do anything alone to mild discomfort when exerting yourself. For some women pains are intermittent and stabbing, for others they are a dull ache that become sharp pain with sudden movement. In either case sudden movement can make them more acute. If you have a difficult labour before a caesarean you may experience pain in more areas. In most cases expect to feel sore towards the end of each pain management period in the first 24 hours. Pain levels decrease over the next few days and unless you develop an infection or other complication you should be free of pain relief medication within 7-10 days. The need for pain relief is less likely when recovering from a *straightforward* vaginal birth.

"If I've learned anything in ten years of motherhood, it's that the way our children are brought into the world means very little for how they live in the world. Nor do the intense hours in which we become mothers shape the months, years and decades of our actually being mothers. And if the experience of childbirth is in fact a crucial process, then let it be the process of teaching us that our children will emerge in ways varied and complicated, not necessarily in times or manners of our choosing, neither made in our image nor as proof of our prowess. Let birth remind us that, with children, so little goes according to even the most well-drawn plan." Tova Mirvis, Mother[129]

Tiredness

You are likely to feel worn out after disturbed nights during pregnancy followed by the emotional and physical upheaval of birth, even more so if you have laboured before a caesarean. Regional anaesthetic does *not* tend to make you drowsy though with a general anaesthetic lethargy can last up to 24 hours.

Blood loss (lochia)

The amount of vaginal blood loss varies and happens even after a caesarean. Initially the blood will be bright red and you may need to change a maternity pad every hour. This slows and gradually becomes dark brown. Avoid tampons for a couple of weeks to reduce the likelihood of infection.

Abdominal cramps

These can be very painful (similar to labour pain) though some women only feel mild twinges. These are contractions helping your uterus return to shape and tend to be stronger when breastfeeding.

Abdomen size

You will still look 7 month's pregnant after delivery but bloating decreases over the next few days. Overall weight loss will take longer.

The incision:

- **Falling out** – It can feel like your insides might fall out. Pregnancy has stretched your stomach muscles and after birth everything feels like it is dropping. After vaginal birth the sensation can feel like everything is falling out of your

> *"I was very disappointed with the size of my tummy after S was born. I had just assumed once he was out I would look back to normal. I couldn't believe I still looked 6 months pregnant." Lucy (31)*

bottom and after a caesarean more like *through* the incision. In both instances this is not actually going to happen, internal stitches are very strong. As muscle tone improves the sensation will disappear

- **Blood loss** – In most instances the incision seals before you remove your bandage. But it is equally normal for a small amount of bleeding to occur from the skin edges, especially if clips or staples have been used. Get it checked, but it will usually stop with a few minutes pressure on the skin edges. If you notice significant blood loss or weeping from your incision seek advice immediately as it may indicate infection

- **Puffiness** – As normal bloating decreases you may notice puffiness around the incision. In many cases this gradually decreases. It can take several months and for some may never entirely disappear, particularly if excess weight remains. Overexertion can cause it to last longer

- **Numbness** – A numb sensation can continue around the incision and/or epidural site after the anaesthetic has worn off. This may be total numbness or a tingly feeling. For most women this entirely disappears within a few weeks but for some it can take six months and for a few women *normal* sensation, in small patches, may never completely return

- **Sharp incision twinges** – These are similar to those experienced by women recovering from an episiotomy and vaginal tear repairs. They are generally caused by overexertion or careless movement, so avoid sudden movements and heavy lifting. You will quickly learn what causes it in your case (e.g. twisting or lifting)

- **Tightening** – The incision may feel tight. This is common to any healing as your skin knits back together and will be experienced after a vaginal birth if there are cuts or tears

- **Itching** – As the incision heals it is common, again as for any cut or abrasion, for it to feel itchy. If this is accompanied by fever, chills, fluid or dizziness seek advice as it may indicate infection. If you feel itchy all over it may be dehydration accompanying the onset of breastfeeding so drink more water

Breast aches and pains

You will probably experience a dragging sensation in your breasts as your milk comes in, irrespective of whether you choose to breastfeed or not. Known as *letdown*, it often coincides with your baby's cry. Once breastfeeding is established, even other baby's cries can cause the milk to flow, so have breast pads easily accessible.

Trapped gas

This can be very uncomfortable. Constipation and trapped gas are natural side effects of pregnancy exacerbated by anaesthetic and, in the case of a caesarean, longer periods of immobility.

Nausea

A general anaesthetic can make you nauseous, whilst regional anaesthetics rarely do. This should disappear as it wears off.

Practicalities

There are lots of practical things you can do to relieve and manage post-birth sensations, significantly improving your recovery. Some simply make your life easier, but others are crucial for ensuring your body is given time and space to recover quickly and efficiently. Many of the suggestions apply equally well to vaginal birth. Not all will feel right for you. Try things out, adapt them and ignore the rest.

Pain management

Once back on the ward you will be given additional pain relief. Understand your schedule (how much and how often) and follow it rigorously. Delays cause pain build-up and stop you feeling able to move about or sleep properly, delaying your recovery. Research suggests that if you fall behind with medication, even by 20 minutes, your ability to *catch-up* is affected and you may experience unnecessary pain. Staff can be busy and may not always keep to the strict schedule that is necessary so keep an eye on the clock. A timely but pleasant request can help keep you on track. Pain relief can mask discomfort so take care when moving about. If you are

> **Keep medication on track**
>
> "Taking your pain medication at regular [safe] intervals, before the previous dose has a chance to wear off, will allow you to stay ahead of the pain" Maureen Connolly, Birth Commentator [130] et al

breastfeeding keep an eye on the condition of your nipples and use barrier creams if necessary.

Looking after your baby

It is entirely possible to pick up and care for your baby after a caesarean. You may not rush to her side the moment she makes a peep but the same is true for some women recovering from a vaginal delivery. This phase is very short lived and staff and your birth partner are available to help. Have your baby's cot placed next to the head of your bed with a leg gap between and the brake on. Have all items you may need in easy arms reach. Alternatively, keep her with you on the bed. Staff may help you create a safe space. However, hospital policy may state that you cannot sleep with your baby on your bed so if you fall asleep while feeding or cuddling do not be surprised to find that she has been moved back to the bassinette.

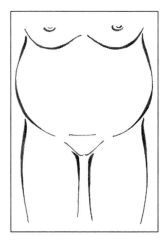

Figure 2 - Typical incision position

Incision care

Assuming all is well you will be asked (after 12 hours approx.) to remove the bandage. Have clean hands to avoid wound infection. Pressure bandages are sticky round the edges and so easier to remove in the shower. You may not be able to bend to see the incision clearly so use a mirror if necessary. Talk to staff beforehand so you know what form of closure technique has been used, metal staples can be a shock otherwise. Typically the incision is 20cm long and a slightly raised, horizontal red or pink line along your bikini line (see Figure 2). Look at your incision, you need to recognise changes. An increase in redness, weeping and/or puffiness or if you have a raised temperature may indicate infection.

- Follow care instructions – these may vary depending on the type of closure technique used and whether or not the wound has healed. It is very rare for an incision to re-open but the surface layer may if you move around too soon and too vigorously

- Initially the area may look bruised, red and irritated or the wound may quickly become a thin red line. The scar vividness will decrease and can be a barely discernable fine white line within months. Where complications arise (e.g. infection), healing may take longer. The residual scar varies according to: skin type, excess weight, your diet etc. Vitamin E and arnica *may* help keep your skin supple, stimulate blood circulation, reduce inflammation and relieve itching, however these are not clinically proven for use in this situation. Such treatments will not remove the scar but *may* improve it

Going to the toilet

Your catheter remains in place for up to 12 hours, longer if there are bladder complications. Going to the toilet for the first time can be daunting whether you have had a vaginal or caesarean birth. For different reasons you may be worried about the strain it will place on parts of your body. To reduce the *worry* of the first few trips try some or all of the following:

- Get help walking to the toilet

- Cradle your incision to make it feel more secure when walking and sitting

- Do not rush and strain. Remain seated for a few minutes if nothing is happening rather than giving up immediately. Try leaning backwards rather than hunching forward and wriggle around a little, without straining

- Move around frequently during the day to keep your digestive system working and relieve trapped gas. Drink plenty of water, eat fruit or try peppermint tea to reduce trapped gas, prune juice for constipation and camomile tea is recommended by some as useful in combating uterine cramps

Constipation

This can be alleviated by drinking fluids (peppermint tea in particular) and eating fruit. If severe, medication is available but do not self-medicate with laxatives. Walking around the ward is actually the most effective way of getting your systems moving again.

Blood clots

Keep your DVT stockings on till you leave hospital. Do gentle ankle rotations and leg movements to reduce the possibility of clots forming (see Figure 3 & Figure 6).

Itchiness

As your incision heals it may itch. Avoid scratching. Mild creams can reduce irritation but only use these with supervision and *not* on an open wound. Itching on arms and legs can coincide with the onset of breastfeeding due to dehydration so drink plenty of water. When showering only use soap on skin that is *obviously* dirty. Soap removes natural oils that protect the skin. Dry yourself carefully but avoid excessive rubbing, a hairdryer set to *cool* is the best way to dry yourself between your legs without irritating the skin if you have *damage* there too. If your vagina or nipples are itching this may be thrush so seek advice as you and your baby will need to be treated.

Nausea

Eat light snacks and drink *non-fizzy* drinks despite the nausea if you can. This will help to keep your strength up, important not only for your own recovery but also for the development of your breast milk.

Moving

There are good reasons for moving about as early as possible. Walking improves circulation reducing the risk of blood clots and stimulates your digestive systems, reducing the chance of severe constipation:

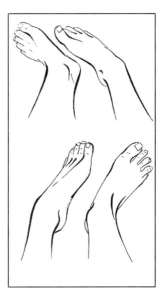

Figure 3 – Ankle rotations

- Plan your movement and activities before you do them. This sounds like overkill but in the first day or so, movement is likely to be your primary difficulty. By minimising sudden movements you can manage the discomfort more effectively

- Do not expect too much of yourself, take notice of warning twinges

- Understand where you are in your pain relief schedule and do not try anything unless the pain is under control. If someone is insisting you get up, only do so when your next round of medication has taken effect

- Gentle ankle rotations ensure you will not have numb feet when you first stand (see Figure 3)

- Get out of bed by placing forearms and hands beside you on the bed and roll onto your side. Move your legs over the side of the bed and slowly push up (more arms and legs, less abdominal muscles) into a sitting position (see Figure 4). The bassinette should already be close to the bed and everything you need next to you so sit or rest against the bed while you look after your baby. Sometimes a small footstool next to the bed can help (or ask for the bed to be lowered the first time you try to get up). There should be no need to stand unaided

- You may want company the first few times you walk in case of dizziness. Go at your own pace. You may find you hunch over or hold your incision. If this makes you feel better, do it, but it is not necessary and ideally you should walk as straight as possible. Everything will feel rather tight but stitches will not snap

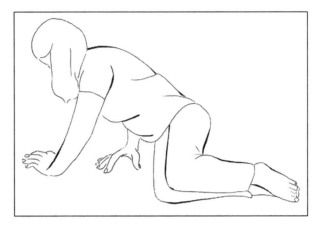

Figure 4 – How to get out of bed

Coughing, sneezing and laughing

These can be painful but cradling your lower abdomen in your hands or pillow can help. If you have had a general anaesthetic you need to clear your lungs regularly. A couple of times an hour take a deep inhalation followed by a full exhalation making an *oof* sound as you do so rather than coughing repeatedly.

Getting enough rest

Nap whenever possible. Headphones (with relaxing music) or earplugs can deaden noise from the ward. Other visitors are not always considerate so if you are having difficulties raise this with staff rather than tackling it yourself. Emotionally you may not be at your best and confrontation may require energy better reserved for looking after your baby. Most hospitals have private rooms available for a small fee that are quieter, giving you time, privacy and space with your new family.

Advice from others

It is a good idea to listen to advice but evaluate it for yourself. Some things are definitely a matter of opinion e.g. the best position to feed in (and later whether or not to use dummies, when to wean etc.). Opinions may be contradictory and this can be rather confusing, particularly in the early days as you get used to your baby. It is important you listen to both what your own body and your baby's are telling you.

Visitors

Restrict the number of visitors and the length of their visit. Of course everyone wants to see and cuddle your baby but think carefully about who really needs to meet her on day one. It can be distressing and exhausting for her to be passed around and handled. Going forward, while newborn babies have your antibodies and so can deal with the *bugs* you may pass on to her, other family members (and especially unrelated visitors) can carry bugs to which she will have little or no resistance. Limiting the number of people handling her for those first weeks/months can help protect her until she develops a more competent immune system. In this first instance, ask your birth partner to manage a visitor schedule agreed in advance rather than trying to do it yourself.

Manage sibling visits carefully. Depending on their age, they will only want to poke, prod and hold your baby for so long and then they will need to be handled sensitively while the visit continues. Have the person who brings them also bring appropriate toys. Remember too that your baby gets lots of presents so a new colouring book or toy for their older sibling can help alleviate initial jealousy. If you feel able to, remind visitors to make a fuss of both baby and sibling(s).

Breastfeeding

It can be difficult and painful establishing feeding whatever type of birth experience you have. For some women breastfeeding is an integral part of caring for their baby, for others it does not feel like an option. Breastfeeding can be highly rewarding with significant medical benefits. For you, it stimulates uterus contractions, helps reduce excess weight gained during pregnancy and facilitates valuable skin-to-skin time strengthening your bond with your baby. For your baby, breast milk contains valuable antibodies and nutrition not found in formula milk and helps kick start her immune system. It can also be very soothing and reassuring for you both. The skin-to-skin and eye contact that naturally occurs during feeding improves your bond, reduces crying and increases the likelihood of successful breastfeeding as well as improving her ability to regulate her own breathing.[131]

Try not to worry if your milk does not come in straight away. It does not mean you cannot feed, just that you may need a bit more support and perseverance.

Get help with how to do it well. It is important that your baby is latched on properly. Put as much of the breast behind your nipple into her mouth as possible. During breastfeeding milk runs from the secreting glands into a set of collecting chambers under the areola (the brown bit around the nipple), your baby doesn't just suck she squeezes these ducts and squirts milk into her mouth.

A caesarean does *not* prevent you breastfeeding.[132] In most cases the amount of pain relief given is so small the effect on your baby is negligible. However, changes to stress hormones as a result of *any* type of traumatic birth (including protracted labour, instrumental birth or unplanned caesarean) can delay lactation.[133] [134]

> *"Regarding breastfeeding advice, you will hear different ideas. Try things out and see what works for you and your baby rather than sticking to the first thing you are told."* Christa Greenacre, NCT teacher (retired)

For some women birth trauma strengthens their determination to breastfeed, for others it becomes associated with the trauma and is not continued.[135]

If you want to breastfeed there are a few things that may make this easier:

- Make use of the support offered by hospital experts. They can help you get comfortable and show you how to latch your baby on, express milk etc.

- Feed regularly. Frequent feeds help establish a good milk supply. At this early stage more frequent feeds are higher in fat/calories – excellent for your baby. There are also lots of useful antibodies in your milk that help to prevent gastroenteritis (bowel infection). The very first milk (colostrum) is especially rich in antibodies. Follow your baby's schedule rather than trying to define one. You can attempt to feed in theatre assuming neither of you are in difficulty. In the case of a general anaesthetic temporary, sensitive use of supplementary feeding techniques (e.g. spoons of formula) can reduce the impact of pain medication[136] and drowsiness

- Padding over your incision helps protect you from wriggling feet. A folded towel or thin cushion is sufficient. Many women do not need this but an infected incision can be particularly uncomfortable

- Get comfortable before starting – you may be feeding for some time so use lots of pillows and perhaps put a cardigan on

- Manage your pain medication properly. This can reduce discomfort in your breasts enabling you to relax more

- Consider using a barrier cream on your nipples to reduce some of the cracking and discomfort sometimes associated with the early stages of breastfeeding

- Try alternative feeding positions more suited to caesareans (see Figure 5). While the cradle position works for many women following a caesarean, *side-lying* puts you and your baby on your sides next to each other and your incision is less easily kicked. Bed-sharing makes it easier to get into position and respond more quickly to the feeding needs of your baby. In the *football* hold you sit up holding your baby to one side rather than across your body again protecting your incision. Lots of pillows can make this position very comfortable. It is easier for managing your baby's latch as you have both arms free

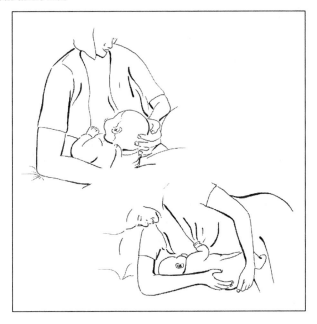

Figure 5 – Breastfeeding positions

- Do not allow your baby to just *chew* on your nipple. Babies like to do this but it can damage the skin of the nipple and cause cracking which is both painful in itself, but increases the likelihood of infection. If your baby likes to chew, give her a clean finger instead

- Keep trying (if you feel able to). Trauma can delay lactation so persevere if you feel able. If your baby's weight is becoming a concern discuss options. Trained lactation specialists can advise you on the best way to give milk to your baby with other devices (syringes, cup feeding, finger feeding and eye-droppers) to avoid subsequent nipple rejection. Bottle teats, for example, can have a detrimental effect on later breastfeeding[137] while using a spoon does not. The reason for this is that your baby is likely to find a bottle teat much easier to get milk from and so rapidly

> **Side-lying**
>
> This can feel a little strange as your muscles will not stop everything feeling like it is *dropping*, balling two muslins under your belly can reduce the sensation until muscle strength improves.

learns to prefer this form of feeding, so always integrate bottles with care. They can be a great way for Dad to have time with his baby

- Be patient. It can take several weeks to establish a successful routine and for the discomfort to disappear. Seek out local support groups if you feel that would be helpful (see Other resources)

- If your baby is in SCU you can express milk for her (having her picture in front of you can help stimulate *letdown*). Continuing to express milk helps prevent your supply dwindling. With care your breast milk can be stored until your baby needs it. If necessary ask for help with breast pumps

- If you are bottle-feeding have someone else make this up and bring it to you. Getting to the kitchen area while holding your baby is probably going to feel daunting in the first day or so. This is not because you cannot carry your baby but rather because it is difficult for you to manoeuvre yourself back into bed and into a comfortable feeding position while holding your baby and the bottle

- Make use of local and national support groups who can work with you as you continue feeding once you leave hospital (see Other resources)

Personal hygiene

To manage blood loss you will require special, longer, thicker sanitary towels. Disposable pants are useful too – size *large* as they do not stretch well. They may not look great but can be thrown away when accidents happen. The high waistline is above your incision so should not rub. Naturally you want to freshen up, but you are unlikely to want to get out of bed in the first few hours so wipes are useful. After 12 hours you will be encouraged to shower. Co-ordinate this with topped up pain medication and visitors who can look after your baby so you are not tempted to rush. Perhaps avoid washing your hair on the first day, it is not impossible but lifting your arms above your head may put added strain on your stomach muscles when balancing (some showers do have plastic chairs).

Help

Ask for help if you are experiencing discomfort and feel you cannot manage. In the first 24 hours make sure your buzzer is within reach so that you can call for help without having to get out of bed. If you feel unsteady on your feet ask for assistance reaching your baby, getting to the toilet or back into bed. If you are exhausted staff may, if asked in quiet moments, look after your baby to give you a rest. Do make sure you agree with them what you want them to do if your baby needs a feed while you are asleep.

Keep your strength up

Snacks are essential to keep your strength up. Depending on when your caesarean occurs you may arrive back on the ward between meal times. Light snacks and drinks can supplement hospital food. Drink plenty of liquids to counteract the dehydrating effect of surgery and breastfeeding. You should not be thinking about getting back into shape while in hospital. However ankle circles (see Figure 3) and calf stretches (see Figure 6) help keep the blood flowing in your legs reducing the chance of blood clots. Gently rocking back and forth occasionally will help your digestive system too. Later, regular pelvic floor exercises (Kegels – see Figure 7) are a good habit and will help reduce urine leaks when laughing or coughing and may prevent uterine prolapse etc. [More Info.[ix]]

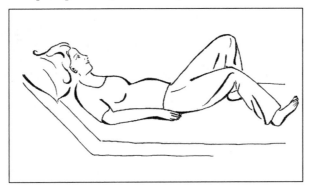

Figure 6 – Leg slide

Pain medication

Do not leave hospital until you have all the pain and constipation medication you require. There should be enough to last you a couple of weeks.

Passing the tests

Before leaving hospital, practitioners will look for signs that you are both ready to go home e.g. a good established feeding pattern, that your bowels are moving properly.

Only leave when you are ready

A typical hospital stay after a caesarean is 2-3 days. You can even be discharged the day after the caesarean if there are no on-going

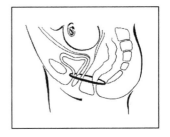

Figure 7 – Pelvic floor muscles (indicated by dark circle)

[ix] www.patient.co.uk (search for pelvic floor excises)

concerns. While home may be quieter and your *things* around you, it may not be more relaxed. In hospital you have time to dedicate to yourself and your baby without distractions. At home the demands of siblings and visitors will be more difficult to manage. Question why you are being asked to leave if you do not feel ready to do so. If you go home early, go straight home and rest. *Do not* be tempted to go home via the supermarket.

Services

Understand the support network in your area and who will check on you e.g. the midwife and health visitor network. You may also want to ask about breastfeeding clinics and mother and baby groups in your area.

De-brief

Request a full de-brief of your delivery or agree when it will take place if you do not feel ready. Not all hospitals offer this service automatically. It is important you understand the circumstances around your caesarean, particularly an unplanned one. This can be highly relevant to future births and may also help you come to terms with your experience. You may want to request your delivery notes too (retrospectively there can be a charge for this).

Getting home

Have your baby's car seat installed in advance and take a baby blanket and cap to protect her from the elements. Use a small towel or cushion between your lower abdomen and the seat belt for your journey home. The driver should take corners more slowly as your stomach muscles will not be strong enough to hold you comfortably in your seat.

Don't over do it

Once home it is tempting to do too much too soon. If your caesarean has been straightforward you will be able to walk and move about with relative ease. *Do not over do it.* View twinges as a warning to slow down. The last thing you want is to be back in hospital because the incision is bleeding or infection has set in.

Maintain your pain medication schedule

Keep strictly to the pattern set, even as your condition improves. It is unlikely you will feel able to drop the medication for at least 7 days. Perhaps set an alarm, even during the day.

Keep checking your incision

Check your incision each day. If necessary, seek advice if you feel any changes do not look or feel right.

Your nest

At home ensure those places where you spend most of your time are comfortable and contain everything you are likely to need so you are not constantly going up and down stairs (see Chapter 5).

Ask for help

The first few weeks can be emotionally and physically draining. Ask for help from others if you feel that would benefit you. You may need help for longer if you have other siblings at home. Friends can come over to cuddle your baby for an hour while you have a nap. Ask people to cook dinner or do the washing/ironing. Be specific about the help you need and use the time to sleep or relax. If you suspect certain people may expect you to entertain them then ask someone else. Your children can help too. Most enjoy *helping mummy* but for very young siblings perhaps try and turn jobs into a game. It should go without saying that you could thank them and say how proud you are of them and reward their help occasionally.

Moving about

Back at home it is important to keep moving in order to maintain good circulation. Getting in and out of chairs or bed still needs forethought for a time. You will use your hands and arms rather than your stomach muscles so sit/lie where you can safely place your baby while you manoeuvre (see Chapter 5) or have someone take your baby while you get up.

Limit visitors

Of course you want to show off your baby and people want to cuddle and coo but as in hospital, manage how it happens and limit the number. As well as affecting your own rest, studies suggest too many visitors can be disruptive and intimidating for your baby. Some practitioners recommend babies are introduced to no more than 2-3 new people in the first week. An open house works for some people, particularly those confident enough to say "I am off to nap now, see you in an hour", but if you feel unable to do this, arrange specific times for people to visit. Visitors should understand that if they want a cup of tea, they will need to make it themselves and there is nothing wrong with asking them to put your pre-prepared meal in the oven before they leave.

Support from others

You will probably have lots of questions in the first few weeks, health visitors, midwives and relevant organisations are generally available to support you. You should feel able to ask anything from how to best hold your baby in the bath, to checking your

> *"My antenatal class continued meeting up afterwards. It has been brilliant. I have made some excellent friends. I can turn up in whatever state of dress or mind and I am accepted." Jess (28)*

scar or your baby's poo. If they are not helpful or you feel they are too judgemental, try alternative sources. Many communities have *new parent* support groups and breastfeeding groups. Joining one of these can be a great source of information and gives you access to other women at the same stage of motherhood as you. A number of national organisations can provide you with local or telephone support for specific issues (see Other resources).

Rest

For the first few weeks avoid housework and do not lift anything heavier than your baby. Be realistic and slow down for a while. Does it matter if dirty pots remain in the sink overnight or the kids have sandwiches for tea three nights in a row? It will not last forever. Share night-time and evening baby care with your partner and decide who is doing what when your baby wakes. Finally, you may want to sleep slightly propped up for a week or so to make getting out of bed that bit easier.

Sleeping

After a few nights at home assess whether the place you have chosen for your baby to sleep is working out. If getting up to go to a cot in another room is too much, perhaps move her to your room or perhaps bed-share until you are more mobile (though some practitioners will advice against bed sharing).

Bed-sharing

If you have had a drink, are taking medication that can make you sleep heavily or are a smoker you are strongly recommended *not* to sleep with your baby in your bed.

Caring for your baby

By the time you go home you should be recovered enough to care for your baby in every respect. However, you may have difficulty emptying a baby bath (perhaps bathe together), or getting out of bed for the eighth time in one night (perhaps have your partner pass her to you on a few occasions).

Eating and drinking

Hard to imagine, but you will forget to eat and drink on occasions. If you are breastfeeding you are likely to be thirsty and it is important you replace lost fluid. Keep a bottle of water in easy reach. You will pee more but emptying your bladder frequently helps reduce the risk of urinary infections as you recover. Continue to eat more fruit, vegetables and protein to help combat anaemia (which can increase tiredness

Belly supports

These are sometimes used during pregnancy but can be useful after a caesarean too. They offer support when lying on your side and rolling over in bed, but are also firm enough to hold a warm or cold compress to alleviate pain or swelling. Doughnut shaped cushions can relieve pressure on sore vaginal areas.

and headaches) as well as to get your digestive system working and continue to avoid processed food. Freeze meals in advance or arrange for family or friends to drop by with the occasional meal.

The 6 week check

Many women feel relatively back to *normal* by this point, at least as normal as they can be when coping with a newborn while being severely sleep deprived. However, everyone is different and rather than aiming for a particular date, listen to your body and only do what you feel able to. You may want to check your motor insurance specifically. It may be the case that your insurer does not cover you to drive until you have passed your 6 week check. Of those contacted during UK research the majority of insurers recommended you do not drive for 6 weeks after a caesarean but did not state this as a policy requirement. A rule of thumb may be not to drive until you feel in full control of your car and able to do an emergency stop if necessary.

Exercise

Many women wait for their 6 week check before starting exercise, but gentle strolls using a pram or papoose can start once back at home. The key with exercise is to take it steady and stop if you feel any pain. Few post-pregnancy books deal specifically with caesarean recovery (see Other resources). Avoid any recommending sit-ups or exercise involving strain to your abdominal area within the first two months. The muscles running vertically down your body (rectus abdominals) separate during pregnancy and need to knit back together before beginning strenuous exercise. Gentle pilates will strengthen these but only go to a practitioner experienced in post-pregnancy pilates. A short, slow swim is another alternative once your incision has healed over. If you do not feel ready to exercise, and many women do not, just try to keep moving and avoid stooping.

Check your rectus abdominals

Lie on your back with your feet flat on the floor, knees raised. Raise your head and shoulders. Using your flattened fingers feel along your mid-section for a ridge of muscle running down your body just above and on each side of your belly button. If the ridge feels like there is a gap between then *knitting* is not complete and you should continue with mild exercise for a while longer, see Figure 8.

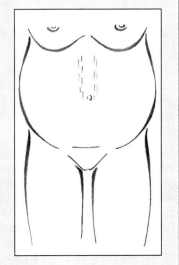

Figure 8 – Rectus abdominals

Continuing hurdles

Pain

In most cases pain should disappear entirely within a month or two of the procedure. If it persists longer seek medical advice. Occasionally adhesions may form connecting tissue internally. This can cause ongoing discomfort and in very rare, severe cases may require further surgery.

Sex

Whether you delivered vaginally or by caesarean, sex may feel impossible both emotionally and physically for weeks if not months. It is generally recommended you avoid sex for 4 to 6 weeks after a caesarean, the same as for vaginal delivery. UK figures[138] suggest the average delay is 8 weeks. In this time incisions and tears should have healed sufficiently, bleeding stopped etc. Some women prefer to wait till after their 6 week check, for others it is a relief to have one part of their life feel a little more *recognisable.*

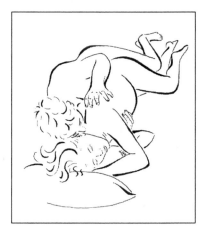

Figure 9 – Spoons position

It is completely normal to be concerned about the first time, particularly if you experienced trauma, physical or emotional. In the case of physical damage to the vagina this may naturally reduce your interest for a time. After a caesarean the abdomen can be sensitive to pressure and twisting actions.

After either mode of birth some women become more interested in sex and others lose interest all together. Varying hormone levels are thought to contribute to this along with tiredness and physical damage. Figures suggest as many as 75% of couples feel their sex life deteriorates for a time.[139] While caesareans will not ensure your sex life is unaffected, evidence suggests it may reduce the chance of pain during sex.[140] Sexual intercourse may also resume sooner than following a vaginal birth.[141] Where severe emotional trauma has occurred it may be worth considering professional counselling. However, all couples, regardless of the delivery they experience, face a time of adjustment, so:

- Take time for yourselves and try to switch off from being mummy and daddy for an hour or two

- Take it at your own pace, do not compare yourself to your friends. You never really know how truthful they are being. Also avoid comparing yourselves to how you were before – you are *both* different now

- Some people find that having a glass of wine can help them relax better

- Use lubrication – breastfeeding mums are particularly likely to be dry. Active breastfeeding suppresses oestrogen levels increasing vaginal dryness (as after the menopause)

- Wear a negligee if you feel unhappy with your current shape, perhaps keep your bra on if you are worried about your breasts leaking at the point of orgasm

- Try different positions. After a caesarean your abdomen may feel tender for a month or more meaning that some positions will feel less appropriate. You may prefer to be on top so that you can control the degree of penetration, or you may find the *spoons* position more comfortable (see Figure 9)

- Always be honest about whether you feel ready or not but bear in mind how your partner is feeling too. Make sure they know you still love them and still find them attractive even if you cannot face sex yet

- Consider alternatives such as oral sex and massage

- Use contraception. The absence of your periods or the fact you are breastfeeding does *not* protects you, you can still become pregnant

- Alter previous habits. Take advantage of your baby's naps, aiming for times when you are feeling more energised i.e. not at the end of a long day of childcare

Your emotional recovery

Whichever way your birth goes it is important to recognise you may experience a range of emotions. These may be anything from euphoria, pride, wonder/awe to mild/severe negative reactions. Most likely is a mixture of all of these.

A new life arriving is an emotional, life-changing experience, even if you have given birth before. In addition to getting to know your new baby you need to get to know the new you. You may not recognise your own body or your emotions. You are likely to be exhausted and may physically feel like you have been hit by a bus. This makes you an easy target for depression, be that mild *baby blues* or postnatal depression.

There is no such thing as a *normal* reaction. Your baby's arrival can leave you with amazing highs and crashing lows. A myriad of factors will effect your emotional recovery: the circumstances of your birth, the health of your newborn, the progress of your physical recovery, hormone levels, how much sleep you are getting, the strength of your preference for a specific type of birth, the amount of support you have afterwards and whether you managed to breastfeed if that was your aim.

Where you are experiencing difficulties early treatment can make all the difference (see Appendix D).

How might I feel?

Many women find a caesarean, planned or otherwise, a powerful, if exhausting, experience and one to remember positively forever. For these women coming to terms with the whole experience can be quite straightforward. In these instances a good bond is often established with relative ease and women can move on to the next stage, that of balancing becoming a mum with being an individual. This in itself is no small feat and one that can inspire a range of emotional reactions too. Motherhood is complex (see Other resources).

> **Emotional reactions**
>
> A study comparing emotional outcomes of each mode of birth found that planned caesareans are likely to have better psychological outcomes for women than instrumental vaginal births and unplanned caesareans.[142]

It is unfortunately the case that for many women unplanned caesareans and medical intervention of any sort leads to negative thoughts and feelings. These can take over and make recovery much more complicated. Feelings of failure and powerlessness can leave you vulnerable and affect your self-esteem. The resulting loss of confidence can significantly affect the way in which *some* women bond with and breastfeed their babies. Try to focus on the positive – your baby has been delivered successfully following a situation where either you and/or she had been at risk. You are not alone, women can feel like this even after a straightforward vaginal birth.

The remainder of this chapter concentrates on recovery from negative emotional reactions as it is in these instances that your health, your bond with your baby and your relationship with partners and siblings can be most affected. Emotional responses are very complex and personal so if need be seek personalised support from skilled practitioners (see Other resources).

> *A mum talking about life after her first caesarean said "My mum and sister alternated staying with us for three weeks after T went back to work. It was brilliant. It took a lot of the stress out of the day, I didn't need to have my eye on the clock for meals and school pick-ups. I couldn't have managed without them." Kerry (31)*

Negative reactions

Emotional trauma should not be underestimated. Even straightforward births can feel difficult, lack of control or a poor relationship with practitioners can feel just as difficult to come to terms with as a medicalised birth. After birth what is interpreted as manageable *baby blues* by one mother may feel totally unacceptable to another, without actually qualifying as postnatal depression (PnD) or post traumatic stress disorder (PTSD). The feelings may last days, weeks or, in the case of PTSD and PnD, years and if not dealt with can affect your ability to *move on*, having knock-on effects on family relationships and even decisions to have other children.

The following list may give you an idea of the spectrum of reactions. You may experience several of the following:

- She arrived and I felt this was the most wonderful experience of my life

- I was overwhelmed with love

- I feel like I have started a whole new, exciting stage of my life

- I sometimes burst into tears for no reason, I am not unhappy I just cry a lot

> *After an unplanned caesarean followed by a planned caesarean a mother said "I felt completely worthless as a mother the first time. I cried all the time and felt I had created a child that cried all the time. I truly believe it [depression] all came from how we started out [unplanned caesarean]. I cannot believe the difference this time. I feel like a different person." Sarah (33)*

- I feel angry that I lost control of my birth, everything happened so quickly I had no opportunity to ask the questions I needed to ask

- I cannot get over the fact my child and I nearly died

- If only I had avoided x or done more y

- My birth did not go anything like to plan, I feel devastated by what happened

- I keep getting flashbacks to being rushed into theatre, the reasons behind the whole emergency are terrifying

- I am grieving the loss of my identity, my body let me down and I feel really angry

- I am confused about the details of what happened

- I do not think my caesarean was necessary, I feel like I have been violated and cheated

- I felt very uninvolved in my birth

...and the list can go on. The point is to show that some triggers are within your control and some are not. Some you will not recognise and others you will be able to relate to. Some you can deal with quite easily, some may need support to come to terms with.

Such reactions are not exclusive to caesareans nor even to very difficult vaginal births so it is useful to understand the spectrum of reactions and possible triggers. Seek help if need be. In mild cases this knowledge may be enough to get you through the few days or weeks of *weepiness* with no extra help. On the other hand you may benefit from additional support in the form of birth de-briefs, counselling etc. See Appendix D for more information about *baby blues,* PnD and PTSD.

> *"Feelings of guilt and sadness surrounding a difficult birth can get in the way of your recovery. Focus on your baby, she knows nothing about your birth plan but wants your attention and needs you to get to know her wishes and feelings for a long time ahead."* Christa Greenacre, NCT teacher (retired)

What can I do to help myself?

Firstly preparation is important (see Chapter 5). Be aware that *narrow* birth plans, poor understanding of medical indications for intervention and inadequate postnatal review[143] [144] all have the potential to negatively affect you (as does the more obvious challenges of medical intervention[145]).

Secondly there are lots of things you can try after your birth to help you in your emotional recovery. The following are some ideas. What works for one person will not necessarily work for another. Bear this in mind and ignore those that do not feel right for you. If you are reading this after the event try not to worry. There are still lots of things you can try.

Bonding

Some women feel an immediate bond with their babies. For others it takes weeks or months. Both are common and *normal*. Do not berate yourself if bonding is not instant, guilt only slows the process. Instead concentrate on caring for your baby and spend lots of quiet time with her. From her point of

> **Understand caesarean birth**
>
> "Mothers generally have a much better experience of operative delivery if they are adequately prepared for it and are supported by staff in terms of being kept informed throughout the whole process. This point is borne out by the fact that women having elective caesareans report greater satisfaction with the operation than those that have had emergency sections." Dr Colin Francome, Emeritus Professor in the Sociology of Health at Middlesex University[146] et al

view everything is probably fine. For some women the process of getting to know their baby, learning how to soothe and care for her is the key to bonding, rather than the *instant love* frequently described as *bonding*. The practicalities of feeding, changing and running around tidying up the minute she goes to sleep can prevent you from just enjoying her, whether she is awake or not, so try to *slow down*. If you feel the bond is really not developing and several weeks have passed seek advice as negative thoughts may be getting in the way, you may need to actively address this.

Talk to others

Sharing the experience and being listened to by someone who understands can really help. Do not be afraid of talking to relative strangers. Birth is one of those experiences that brings people together and knowing you are not alone or unusual can help. There are lots of organisations, books and discussion forums that may suit your specific needs (see Other resources). While it is important you do not shut out your partner and family you need to be aware they can only help so far. If difficult feelings persist you may need to access other sources of support. Some therapists/organisations offer targeted counselling. Your health visitor or doctor should have a list of practitioners in your immediate area. You may require a referral to get things moving but it is worth jumping through the hoops to get to the people you need.

> *A mum talking about her first birth, an emergency caesarean said "It wasn't that I hadn't done it [birth] properly, I just thought oh my poor child, I put him through this. I lost my connection with S, I was too ill and too exhausted. I just couldn't think of him." Sarah (33)*

Find out why you had a caesarean

You were probably told at the time but in an unplanned caesarean it is understandable if you forget the details. You are entitled to a full debrief and most hospitals do this, some automatically, others at your request. It can help you come to terms with what happened as you talk through the whys and wherefores. You may want to delay this for a week or so but do go back to it. Understanding the circumstances and decisions that led to your caesarean is, for some, enough to start healing. Look in detail at how your caesarean actually progressed, the specific order of events. Were there elements you did not understand? This can be anything from why you felt queasy one minute and off in a dream-world the next to why you had a general rather than a regional anaesthetic. It is particularly important to do this as it may have a bearing on your plans for future pregnancies. If you feel a caesarean was performed unnecessarily, it will be understandably harder to come to terms with and a *debrief* alone may not be sufficient.

Evaluate the reason

Once you know the reason(s), ask questions about the specific condition or situation. Perhaps read about it and talk to others who have had the same experience. Some conditions may be easier to come to terms with than others, e.g. knowing your condition was life threatening may reduce disappointment or anger if you can believe your caesarean saved your life. Involve your birth partner – they may have helpful memories but they may also have negative feelings which need tackling in this way too.

Evaluate the experience

Think about how the experience has made you feel about yourself. Think too about how you felt at the time including how you were treated and supported through your birth. Some of the negativity may be related more to interactions with specific members of staff or support at home than the actual caesarean. If so, deal with that separately. Something as simple as a letter to the hospital talking about your experience or a review on a user opinion site e.g. www.patientopinion.org.uk, with suggestions for how it could be improved, may prove quite cathartic.

Grieve

Do *not* bottle up your emotions: grieve for the birth you did not have. Talk about it, write about it, do whatever feels right to help you start to deal with the feelings of loss or disappointment that may have become associated with the arrival of your baby.

Ring the changes

Recognising new experiences for what they are can alter the perspectives you may have developed about them. For example, while you love your baby to bits, sometimes you may feel like an invisible dairy cow as everyone coos over her and practically ignores you. Try thinking instead that she has been excitedly anticipated for months so she will get more attention in the short term. Similarly, while you may feel thrilled about being able to breastfeed you may also feel apprehensive about the physical changes that are happening to your body and breasts as a result. Try thinking instead that you are providing her with the best possible start in life and are successfully fulfilling a key role of motherhood.

Consider breastfeeding

Breastfeeding can be an excellent way to spend quality time with your baby aside from all the health benefits it brings to the both of you (see – this chapter). It can be difficult to establish however so persevere if you feel able to. If you previously decided not to breastfeed but are feeling disappointed about your birth, you may want to think again about

> *A mum reflecting on her first birth said "I am so disappointed with the way I was born [induction and forceps]. I think I will always wonder if I could have done anything differently." Amanda (32)*

breastfeeding. Some women feel it is a second chance at *getting it right*. If it seems it is not going to work for you, try not to blame the caesarean as this only creates more emotional baggage. There are many reasons why women choose to stop breastfeeding: breast infections, painful and bleeding nipples, the baby is not thriving on the breast milk they are getting, medication Mum may require is not safe for the baby etc. So instead allow yourself to grieve knowing you have tried and made an informed decision to stop. Looking further ahead, it may be that you breastfeed for a time and then come to a decision to stop. Sleep deprivation, isolation, lack of support as well as needing to go back to work may contribute to this and again it is important you feel happy with your decision and allow yourself time to acknowledge this phase is passing.

Photographs of your birth

If you have had a general anaesthetic it may help to have someone visit you after surgery to talk about it. If you have planned it in advance this visit can include photographs of your baby being cleaned and checked during her first hour.

Manage your recovery

Get plenty of rest – sleep when she sleeps even if the washing does not get done or tea is late. Set realistic goals for yourself each day. In the beginning goals may be a brief stroll to the end of the street or washing your hair. Caesarean or not you may not feel up to much more than that as you get used to early motherhood.

Write your birth story

Some women find this cathartic, even without showing it to anyone. Sometimes the act of describing incidents and feelings on paper can alter or add a new perspective.

Future births

Research suggests many women, following instrumental (7 in 10) or caesarean (4 in 10) birth, still prefer a vaginal birth for their next child.[147] It is important therefore that you do all you can to understand this birth. When you have your debrief determine whether any issues associated with this caesarean mean you are likely to need a caesarean next time (see Appendix B).

Your emotions, memories and the emphasis you place on these can play a significant part in whether you can face another birth. It is important to deal with any negative emotions this time round to avoid transferring the anxiety and stress to your next pregnancy (see Appendix D).

Your baby's recovery

Many ideas already discussed in this chapter (see also Chapter 5 & Appendix A) will help her recovery just as much as yours e.g. managing visitors, quiet time together, skin-to-skin time and breastfeeding.

In addition consider the following:

Talk to her

She knows your voice well so reassure her you are nearby even if it is by giving a running commentary about what you are making for dinner.

Comforters

When you are absent perhaps place a safe comforter near your baby that smells of you. Alternatively swaddle her in a small blanket that you have slept with for a couple of nights, again the scent will reassure her.

Avoid over stimulation

Save the many mobiles and visual stimulants that arrive as presents until later. She does not need ten teddy bears, two multi-coloured mobiles and a musical box tinkling in the corner right away. The sights and sounds of her new world are just as interesting.

Swaddling

Tightly wrapping your baby can reassure and calm her as it replicates some of the sensation of the womb. Perhaps stop swaddling around 1 month old, or before if she shows signs of always trying to get out, some babies love it, some do not.

Familiar rhythms

Gently patting her to the rhythm of your heartbeat may jog comforting memories from before birth.

Baby massage

This is an excellent way of getting to know your baby and particularly good for helping you become increasingly confident in handling and caring for her. Getting the amount and type of massage right is important so be guided by trained practitioners, such confident physical contact may be reassuring for your baby, but too much can be intimidating. Classes can be fun and a good way of meeting other mums but bear in mind that such environments are noisier and may not suit your baby – using massage at home may be better.

My baby is in the Special Care Unit

When a baby is in the SCU it is a distressing time for everyone. If moving around is still difficult ask for a wheelchair so you can be moved to her as soon as possible. Sensory awareness of your presence contributes significantly to her wellbeing.

Techniques for supporting her are:

- **Scent** – Bring clothing or other small items that you have slept with – they carry your scent and can be placed inside the bassinette / incubator next to her

- **Touch** – Although sick babies can react badly to handling because it disturbs their heart rate and blood pressure, your baby will inevitably be handled a lot because of the amount of attention she needs. What will help is reassuring touch from you. *Still touch* is recommended. Gently place your hand on her and keep it still, she may find stroking too stimulating. Awake or not this helps bonding and reassures her. Watch for reactions of over stimulation and stop when necessary. Only attempt finger tip massage if this has been agreed with her carers and again watch for reactions and respond accordingly

- **Voice** – Talk to her a lot. It does not matter what you say, it is your specific voice that will reassure. She has been listening to you for months already

Remember to look after yourself too. Take breaks and make sure you get enough food and sleep so you are feeling well during the precious time you spend with her. Take one day at a time and celebrate each positive event. You may have sadness, worry and shock to cope with and you may still need to grieve what some term the *ambiguous loss* of a premature or traumatic birth. Talk with your partner and contact support groups dedicated to working with people in your position. Your extended family can help in all sorts of ways (see Chapter 6).

> **Ambiguous loss and the *joy-grief* contradiction**
>
> This term attempts to describe the feeling some parents have when they are unable to express the emotions surrounding the birth of a premature or sick baby. Some feel that they should not be grieving at all because they ought to be experiencing the joy of their baby. Ambiguous loss is very traumatic for all involved. [More info.[x]]

---

[x] Powell KA, 'Ambiguous loss: Experiencing joy and grief after the birth of a premature child' 2001 www.prematurity.org

My baby died

While very rare, this does happen and is understandably very distressing for all concerned. It is very important to grieve the loss of your baby. Everyone grieves in different ways and your extended family will all need time too. While in hospital it is helpful to be transferred to a ward where you cannot hear other new babies. This should be done automatically but if it is not request this if you think it will help you.

Leave-taking is an important part of the grieving process. Everyone has different ways they want to do this. For example, some parents want to spend time with their baby saying good bye, others prefer photographs to be taken by the nursing team. Your hospital will have had experience of this and may be able to make some suggestions that feel appropriate for your specific circumstances. Once back at home you may want to arrange for family and friends to join you in a formal *leave-taking* to recognise the presence of your baby in your life.

There are quite a few organisations aiming to support parents and extended families cope and come to terms with the loss of a baby (see Other resources). If you feel able, it is worth getting in touch with them as they can provide not only a listening ear but also tailored counselling and put you in touch with other families with similar experiences.

My partner's recovery

It is easy to forget your partner in all the upheaval – you will naturally be concentrating on you and your baby. However your partner is experiencing much of the upheaval too and it is helpful and considerate to remember this. Birth, as witnessed by them, can be very difficult. They may need time and support to come to terms with it even if the birth was straightforward. Granted they will not be dealing with physical recovery issues, nor may they be dealing with night-time feeding if you are able to breastfeed. However, they are dealing with a birth experience, getting to know a new baby and witnessing huge changes to you, their life circumstances and the expectations that are now being placed upon them. So give them time to adjust too.

How might they be feeling?

With the best will in the world your partner is unlikely to have read as widely, attended as many classes or talked about birth as much as you have, but they will have formed an impression of what it is going to be like. The extent to which their experience matches their preconceptions will influence the emotional upheaval they will experience.

The extent to which they felt able to be involved in the birth will vary from person to person and may have changed from what was planned in any case. The more comfortable they feel with their overall role the more they are likely to be able to help you going forward. The following are just a few of the natural, *normal* reactions they may be experiencing:

- Excitement at getting to know their new baby

- Euphoria / distress about the things they witnessed during the birth

- Questioning the role they played in the birth

- Confusion at the degree of change that is happening around your home and in your relationship

Paternal postnatal depression (PPnD) is not very well known, but it does exist and the impact of it upon your relationship and children can be significant.[148] Relationship breakdown is quite common in the first year after a birth and evidence suggests that in some cases this may be directly related to Dad suffering postnatal depression.[149] So in the midst of all the upheaval try to take time to think about your partner too. They may be feeling some or all of the following:

Fear

Even the most straightforward birth can be traumatic for the birth partner. Seeing a loved one in pain can be frightening and frustrating. If the birth becomes less straightforward it can be very traumatic: Will my partner be ok? Is the baby going to survive? How much damage is there going to be? How will we cope at home? Is this really necessary? Should I be intervening? It can be particularly stark if you have a general anaesthetic as they will be left standing outside theatre for a time with no feedback on how you or your baby are doing. Their imaginations may run riot and such an experience can raise all sorts of issues for them afterwards.

Lack of control/knowledge

They may feel intimidated by the experts, the situation and their comparative lack of knowledge. They may also blame themselves for not having prevented unwanted intervention. Making decisions on your behalf can add to their stress. For example, unless discussed in advance your partner will, in the case of a general anaesthetic, be making decisions about feeding and clothing your baby for her first few hours. Unless you have discussed it in advance they are unlikely to know what you are planning to do and may not know the potential impact of giving formula instead of breast milk immediately after birth. Try not to criticise decisions, particularly if you did not discuss such eventualities beforehand – they will have done what they thought was right at the time.

Learning on the job

While you are recovering, some jobs you have previously done within the home probably now fall to them. Some may relish this, but others may feel the pressure, particularly if you are overly critical. This will all be in addition to their working day so quite quickly they are going to end up as exhausted as you. Appreciate what they are doing and try not to criticise when things are not done your way. Does it matter if the washing is left in the machine for 24 hours before going into the dryer? Probably not. Nor is it the end of the world if they gave the kids the wrong drinks in their lunchbox.

Sleep deprivation

They are probably going to be almost as sleep deprived as you in the early days so try not to compete over who is most tired, you both are.

Isolation and loss

Your priorities have changed and you may not be communicating as well as before. Try to keep the lines of communication open. You need to be able to talk about what is going on and how you are both feeling. Perhaps consider couple support groups.

How might you appear to them?

When thinking about your birth partner and others close to you, try to bear in mind the following through pregnancy and beyond:

You are probably quite difficult to live with

No doubt you are aware of how much you are changing physically, but you are going to change behaviourally and emotionally too. It is not uncommon for partners to feel like they are living with a different person. For obvious reasons you may become self absorbed, weepy, aggressive, a fanatical nest builder and permanently sleepy (see Figure 10). I am not suggesting you try to revert to your old self – this will feel impossible but do try to remember how different you are going to appear to them and how disconcerting it may be.

> **Competitive exhaustion**
>
> This destructive habit can cause significant problems between couples. Both feel that their daily life is the most difficult and that the other just doesn't understand. They then let resentment fester under the surface or spend valuable time and energy arguing about who has the worse deal. Discuss your day, ask each other for help and support and try to remember that you are *both* going through a huge learning curve while extremely sleep deprived. It is only in truly believing the roles are totally different and have extreme and unique pressures of their own that you can hope to remove this barrier to emotional recovery.

> *A dad reflecting on the antenatal period for their first child said "She seemed to read every birth book there was. I was interested, but really it seemed to go on forever. I felt guilty that I couldn't relate but also resentful that this seemed to be our only conversation for months." Martin (36)*

Keep some perspective

Yes, you are the pregnant one but expecting them to really understand everything is a bit unreasonable. Their hormones are not raging, their body is not changing, so rather than dismissing them for this, view them as your sanity check, your lifeline, and try not to give them a hard time.

Be reasonable

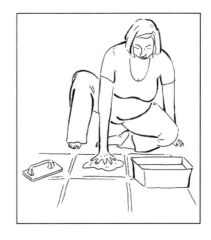

Figure 10 – Grouting the floor tiles

A tub of ice cream at 4am from the all-night store is unreasonable. They too are stressed and their sleep disturbed, after all they may be sleeping next to someone who gets up to pee 4 times a night. You are expecting them to cut you plenty of slack every day so a bit of give and take is important.

If they offer to help, let them

Let them take on more household tasks many partners want to but are not sure what will be the most help. Later when your baby arrives make sure they too have positive time with their baby playing, cuddling and washing etc. They are not just there to take over when your energy has run out or she has been crying for what feels like hours. It is particularly important that they are positively involved early on so they too can feel they are developing a relationship with their baby, they should not feel they are just another pair of hands supporting you.

CHAPTER SEVEN

I am the birth partner, what can I do?

The first thing to say is that I aim to avoid making assumptions about your sex or relationship to Mum. You may be male or female, you may be the father of the baby or not and you may be the person sharing a home with Mum or another friend/family member. As birth partner not only will you be attending the birth but you will likely go on to have a significant role in the baby's care and in the home afterwards. So in this chapter I will refer to the baby as yours and you as *birth partner* irrespective of the subtleties of your actual connection to Mum.

The arrival of your baby is a huge event, if not *the* biggest event of your life so far. The fact that it is not you that is pregnant is unlikely to diminish the magnitude of your feelings.

Culturally, birth partners have come to be defined as *supporters* or *helpers*. For a parent this is rather missing the point, you should be present in your own right to witness the arrival of *your* baby. If you can provide additional support to Mum, great, and it is important that you *both* agree how this is going to work, but you are definitely not there just as a *supporter.*

It is a good idea therefore to begin to develop a sense of what it is you hope to be within your new family. It is unfortunately still the case that some professionals, family, friends and mums are not sure how to treat you during the birth and beyond and unclear about what role you should have. Ideally, the new family learns together with space and time to adjust to family life and importantly with everyone participating on an equal footing.

What is going to happen?

This is the million dollar question. Truthfully it is actually a bit of a lottery. Even a planned caesarean can happen early if Mum goes into labour. The more open minded you both are about the way she gives birth and the more realistic your expectations, the less likely you both are to be disappointed, upset or stressed.

Your antenatal class may have suggested some birth books. Generally written for the mums, these will leave you in no doubt about the details of vaginal birth but will probably do little to prepare you effectively for a caesarean. As with a vaginal birth, take time to understand the practicalities as well as the implications for you (see Appendix A).

What are the practical things can I do?

Before birth

Really it comes down to how you see yourself participating. The following is a list of ideas:

Attend antenatal appointments

Hearing your baby's heartbeat at the scan can be wonderful. It is a perfect opportunity to start learning about your baby first hand. Other appointments can be daunting for Mum and she may want you with her - peeing in a bottle is not stressful but an internal exam may be. If you are present during discussions about birth options you can actively participate in subsequent debate.

> **Learn together**
>
> "Discover that while the male experience of pregnancy is necessarily different from that of the female, it need be neither second-hand nor second class. For there exists a sense in which *both* fathers and mothers are outside looking in, and are building a relationship with a fantasy baby, before its birth." Adrienne Burgess, Head of Research at the Fatherhood Institute[150]

Antenatal classes

Attending these is particularly important if you are going to be the primary birth partner during a vaginal birth. However, many of the things you learn will apply equally well to a caesarean setting. Studies show that men attending antenatal classes feel better prepared for birth and their role in it.[151] Knowing what is going to happen and why can take some of the

> *"I made some really good friends at our antenatal class. The wife of one of the couples in our group had mental health issues, on top of which they were moving house shortly after the birth. All us new dads got together and helped them with the move." Tom (37)*

stress out of the situation. Classes can also introduce you to your own support network - other birth partners. Antenatal classes are not designed to put you on the back foot but they can feel rather alienating being so geared, as they often are, towards Mum. In many cases this is far from intentional and more likely due to a lack of awareness and understanding of the needs and feelings of birth partners. If this is your experience still ask questions, you naturally have needs, worries and questions too and there will certainly be other birth partners in the room with similar thoughts. Some health authorities run classes specifically for expectant fathers, but these are not common.

Understand the birth plan

As birth partner you will hopefully have been involved in its development and are consequently better placed to support and if necessary defend the preferences expressed in it. While Mum is the one physically experiencing labour/caesarean and therefore ought to have significant say in the proceedings, you may have preferences too. It is also quite possible a point may arrive when she is valiantly resisting something that might actually be in her best interests or the baby's. You will need to make sure she is hearing things correctly and can reach an appropriate decision. You are likely to feel more confident in this if you have a good understanding of the issues and her original preference.

> "Looking after a baby is grinding hard work and it helps if there is more than one person around to do it." Marcus Berkmann, writer and father [152]

Paternity leave

If this option is available to you consider taking it. These precious early days with your new baby can be highly rewarding, giving you time to bond with her and develop an understanding of what she needs and how to satisfy these. Bear in mind too that you will be very sleep deprived after her arrival and a week or two to get used to the new *tired* you without the pressure of work can be very useful, to say nothing of the reassurance Mum may get from having you around to share the experience and challenges with.

Face your worries about the birth

If you have concerns try talking things through with someone, not necessarily Mum. It is reasonable and *normal* to have worries, particularly if you have not been through a birth before. Knowing what is going to happen and why it is happening can help (see Appendix A & Appendix B). For some mums your anxiety can make her more anxious [153] so it is important you resolve as much as you can beforehand.

Being at the birth

Being at the birth can be an important shared experience and one to agree between you. You or Mum may not want you there of course and this too needs to be discussed and agreed. Everyone reacts differently and there is no right or wrong position to take. Assuming you are planning to be with Mum expect to see her poked and prodded and naked from the waist down and, at least in the case of a

> **Try to remain calm**
>
> "Caesarean mothers' post-operative pain is strongly linked to their fear-experiences during labour and these [are] mediated by the level of their birth partner's fear." Adrienne Burgess, Head of Research at the Fatherhood Institute [154]

caesarean, in a room full of strangers. Once in theatre a screen will be raised over her chest to obscure the view of surgery. As you will be sitting at her head you too will be unable to see unless you lean around the screen. However it may be that you don't want or are unable to be at the birth, in which case it is a good idea to discuss this possibility ahead of time and jointly decide the alternatives.

Who is your second in command?

Sometimes work commitments or cultural expectations dictate you will not be present at the birth. Or, if your baby comes early, you just may not be able to get there in time. Few babies arrive on their due date, so have a backup plan. It may be that a friend/family member, doula or independent midwife (see Chapter 3) is going to join the two of you in the birth any way in which case they can accompany her in your absence. If you do intend to have additional support with you make sure you agree how the roles are to be divided.

Be ready

Labour can start at any time. From about 8 months onwards avoid being too far away and never drink so much you cannot legally drive. Make sure you know the route – right to the door of the maternity wing, its entrance may be entirely different from the one you have visited for outpatients or A&E. Have a full tank of petrol, know how long the journey takes and keep sufficient coins for the parking meters. In the case of a caesarean you will be taken to gown up and probably brought straight to theatre separately to Mum so if you want to take photos take the camera with you then, you will not have time to nip back for it.

A dad talking about an unplanned caesarean said "I had absolutely no idea what to expect and was told to wait in a room by myself with a silly hat on. I was then led into theatre where my wife lay with various tubes coming from her. That said everything was so calm in the room and the radio was on; I can still remember which songs were playing." Duncan (29)

Pack the bag

You will be fetching and carrying once in hospital. Everything you, Mum and baby need is going to be in *the hospital bag* (see Chapter 5). It will be helpful if you can find everything readily. Also you will be in hospital for hours and you may not have time or want to leave her that often so include things for you too: drinks/snacks, newspaper/book (planned caesareans can become very delayed by other people's emergencies), loose change for the parking meter and phone etc.

Car seat

Sort out the buying and fitting of the seat before the due date. This is particularly important if you are planning a vaginal birth (if Mum is discharged the same day you are unlikely to have an opportunity to go home for it). Without pre-fitting you may find that the first chance you get to do this is when everyone is standing in the lobby waiting for you.

Stay healthy yourself

Consider stopping smoking and establish healthy eating habits, both to encourage Mum during her pregnancy but also to create a healthy atmosphere (literally) at home before your baby arrives. The negative impact of smoke and alcohol in the home both before and after birth is staggering. [More info.[xi]]

During caesarean birth

Breathing

Slow your breath and encourage Mum do the same, she will tend to copy you if you can hold her attention. This can help calm you both.

Take care of yourself

It is not uncommon to feel that you are not making much difference during labour or surgery. Remember your presence alone is very supportive to Mum but more particularly remember that you are there to witness the birth of your baby and that this is a perfectly valid thing to be doing in itself.

> **Benefits of your support**
>
> "Labouring women benefit when they feel *in control* of the birth process... a key component in this is experiencing support from their partner during the birth." Adrienne Burgess Head of research at the Fatherhood Institute[155]

Skin-to-skin with your baby

Your baby will be delivered within the first 10 minutes of surgery. One of you can hold her skin-to-skin. This close contact is very calming and reassuring for her. Research suggests that close contact from you is as positive as from Mum, so much so that your baby may cry less and sleep sooner than babies who are placed in a cot.[156] If you want to do this do not wear a t-shirt/shirt under your theatre gown.

[xi] 'Maternal and infant health in the perinatal period: the father's role Literature Review' undertaken by: Adrienne Burgess at www.fatherhoodinstitute.org

Extra hands

Mum can hold the baby on her upper chest even during surgery and may want to breastfeed in this position. You will probably want to help with this as lying prone means she may not feel confident doing it unaided.

Talk

If Mum is unable to hold your baby in theatre, hold her nearby and talk to Mum about her. It does not really matter what you say, a stream of consciousness will give her a pretty good picture. In the moments when your baby is taken to one side for the various checks, you can go with her and if you do tell Mum what is happening, this can be incredibly reassuring, particularly during an unplanned caesarean where the baby may have been in some difficulty and need immediate support.

Photos

If you have decided to be in charge of the camera during surgery, confirm where you can go in the room before getting up.

Immediately after birth

Baby time

You will be *allowed* to stay with your new family for quite some time, but unfortunately in many hospitals you will not be able to stay over night. Hospital policies tend to exclude birth partners after visiting hours and this can feel particularly harsh where there is a delay in bringing your baby home as in the case of delayed feeding, a caesarean (2-4 days) or an SCU stay. This policy can be very hard to cope with and may have influenced your decision on where to give birth (see Appendix F). Naturally you will want to care for your baby in hospital and there is plenty of opportunity for this, even more so if Mum has had a caesarean. Mum is likely to find moving around rather daunting so it will be easier for you to do some things. This early contact helps many birth partners bond with their baby and it develops more quickly.[157]

Grooming

For some mums how they look is the last thing on their mind, for others the sooner they freshen up the better. Raising her arms after surgery and with an IV still attached means some tasks can actually be difficult initially and she may appreciate your help. So, if she wants it, brush her hair, fetch a damp flannel etc. In many cases she will be expected to have a shower within the first 12 hours and this may seem a huge task to her so she might need your assistance.

Looking at the scar

Mum will be encouraged, if everything is straightforward, to remove the bandage within 12 hours. She will find bending difficult and her stomach will still be quite distended so she may want you to tell her what it looks like. To prepare for this find out what has been used to close the incision as dissolvable stitches will look quite different from metal staples.

> *A dad reflecting on his experience following the birth of his first daughter said "I found I was good at quite quickly was working out why our daughter was crying, it was enormously satisfying to then be able to do the cuddling and changing to make her happy." Simon (38)*

Re-stock supplies

In some cases hospital food is not great, nor served at a time convenient to you. So have a steady supply of snacks and drinks for you both.

Back at home

Get to know your baby

Spend as much time as you can holding and playing with your baby. Bottle-feed her too if this is being used to complement or has had to replace breastfeeding. Paternity leave, if you have taken it, will very soon come to an end so try not to get shoehorned into being solely the chief cook and bottle washer during this time. You need time with your baby too and not just at 2 am when she has been screaming her head off for an hour. Perhaps take on bath-time and turn it into play-time, bending over a bath will be particularly difficult for Mum in any case. Research clearly shows that early involvement before and after birth increases self

> *"During the pregnancy I felt quite disconnected so once E arrived there was finally something to do. It was terrifying of course, because nothing can really prepare you for it, and the sleep deprivation quickly hit us both. While I could not feed her I could do everything else. After a while I found I was quite good at bouncing our daughter in a certain way that helped her go to sleep, then I felt a lot more relaxed." Simon (38)*

confidence and can "improve the father-child attachment, mother-child involvement and breastfeeding rates" (Working with Men group[158]).

Breastfeeding

Encourage breastfeeding but remember that with the best will in the world, some women find prolonged attempts very stressful, so if Mum or baby really cannot take to it, then support her in her decision to stop.

Work commitments

Try to minimize your work obligations so that together you can spend time getting used to being a family. Long work hours can contribute to a pattern of *ships passing*. As Mum gets to the end of her energy each day she may feel she needs to simply hand the baby over to you as you walk through the door and head in the opposite direction leaving little time for you as a couple.

> **Agree roles**
>
> Agree the type of support you feel comfortable with giving "Some fathers don't like the *busy* work assigned to them during their paternity leave, feeling it is a contrived way to make them feel important and included." Penny Christensen, Birth Trauma Canada

Household chores

In the first few weeks Mum will be unable to push a vacuum around, carry heavy shopping or lift siblings out of the bath. You will need to do these things to avoid straining her incision, thereby delaying recovery.

Baby blues or postnatal depression

Despite the euphoria often associated with the arrival of a baby, mums can be really down after the birth. If severe, *baby blues* can be quite distressing and debilitating. Postnatal depression (PnD) is quite another matter however and will need treatment (see Appendix D). If PnD goes untreated it can have a serious effect on your relationship and Mum's ability to bond with her baby. Some partners "experience fear, confusion and a sense of helplessness that they are unable to help their partner overcome their depression" (Post and Antenatal Depression Association[160]) so get support for yourself too. For some, Mum's symptoms can become impossible to live with and this may increase the chance of you becoming depressed too (see Appendix D).[161] If you suspect

> **Give yourself time to learn**
>
> "Many fathers see play as the primary means of developing a close and loving relationship with their children. So when confronted with a tiny baby, many new fathers draw back, unable to work out how to *play* with them or to see another role for themselves. Fathers could be helped to broaden the notion of *play*, [by understanding] that for babies *play* and *care* can be indistinguishable: much play happens during nappy changes, feeding, bathing and so on." Working with Men group[159]

PnD in either of you (yes birth partners can have it too) talk to your health visitor and get help.

Encouragement

In her effort to look after her baby Mum may forget to look after herself so gentle reminders to: nap, drink water and take a short stroll to get some fresh air and keep her circulation going will help.

What might be going on for me?

You will probably have heard a lot about birth and the aftermath from friends and the media, some concentrating on the wonder of it all, others telling you about the baby vomit and the sleep deprivation and all probably telling you to kiss goodbye to your sex life. But here are a few other things to be aware of.

Changing world

From the moment you discover a new life is on the way things begin to change. For many birth partners this is a very exciting time, full of plans and expectations about the baby and the future. The changes in Mum and the home feel positive ones and something to be actively involved in.

Naturally changes can also cause moments of worry for both of you. Trying to identify what it is about the changes that is causing concern means that in many cases you can work out ways to reduce or remove the worry altogether. Fairly common concerns for birth partners revolve around self-doubt and fear of incompetence. Do *not* subscribe to the idea that Mum somehow knows more or is better at caring for her baby than you. You are no less naturally programmed to *know stuff* than she is (see – this chapter). The first time round you are both going to feel pretty clueless at times and you cannot predict every eventuality. Allow yourself to make mistakes and don't castigate yourself for getting it wrong sometimes, there is a lot to learn with each child you have.

> ### Get back on the horse
>
> "Very often when fathers withdrew [from doing things for their baby] it was because they felt incompetent...the more fathers withdraw the more their partners *pick up the slack* ...and the more incompetent the fathers feel, the more they withdraw ... and so the vicious circle continues" Adrienne Burgess, Head of Research at the Fatherhood Institute [162]

Of necessity, getting to grips with caring for your baby takes over for a time. The learning curve for first time parents is particularly steep. It is easy to forget each other in the process and it will take particularly enlightened friends and family to remember it is not all about baby and Mum. In actively participating in the pregnancy, birth and afterwards you can participate in the changes, influence them and get to know your baby in your own way.

Who is this person?

Aside from the size of her belly there may be noticeable emotional changes in Mum. You may feel she's a moving target. Her hormones, priorities and worries may make her unrecognisable at times and this can make it impossible to know what to do for the best at any given moment. You may have found a way through this potential minefield, but if not then being *open and honest* about each other's needs, hopes and fears is a good start.

At first changes may be subtle but she may become increasingly self-absorbed. At times she will be amazed and occasionally horrified at some of the things she is experiencing. Her body and mind are increasingly unrecognisable to her in more ways than the bump and the morning sickness. Her teeth may wobble, her skin and hair change and this may be nothing compared to the emotional rollercoaster she is on. She may cry at TV adverts or tiny shoes in shop windows and she probably knows her reaction to you leaving the milk on the kitchen counter was over the top. Reading the earlier chapters relating to her physical and emotional challenges during pregnancy and recovery may help explain what is happening (see Chapter 1 & Chapter 6 & Appendix D).

She may be rather negative at times. The term *morning sickness* is a bit of a misnomer as she can feel and be sick at any time of the day or night for months with the strain affecting her overall mood, resulting in tears, anger, resentment or just plain confusion.

Expect to talk about all sorts of bizarre details. Each conversation she has or birth book she reads can produce more ideas for her birth that may impact significantly upon you. For example, perhaps she wants photographs of the birth. This is possible but you may be worried what you might see, particularly in a caesarean. Discussing it means you can work out a middle ground ahead of time, e.g. getting agreement from the hospital for a student to take the photos for you. Talk through each other's issues to prepare as best you can.

Am I a loose part or a significant cog?

The quick answer is a significant cog. However with a caesarean birth the room is full of people, all with specific jobs to do and you may feel that with nothing to do you are a loose part. In reality you could view it as you are present as a parent, witnessing the birth of your child and that is significant in itself.

> *"Holding my baby skin-to-skin in theatre was the first time I felt I had done anything in the whole process. It was a tremendous feeling that words cannot really express." Richard (36)*

The practicalities of vaginal birth are such that birth partners are often expected to provide support and opportunities for this are more obvious than for a caesarean birth. That said, do not underestimate the power of your physical presence. As already discussed your presence is incredibly reassuring and you are both likely to view the birth more positively if you have been a positive part of the experience.[163] You can do this just by being present, but for practical ideas see earlier in this chapter.

If Mum is particularly focused on avoiding a caesarean she may not be able to think straight or feel able to make decisions once in labour, so understanding when a caesarean is necessary and when it is still only a recommendation is an important part of being a birth partner. The better informed you are the more you can participate in the discussions (see Appendix B) potentially influencing the direction the birth takes.

Understanding the birth plan and the significance of each point is invaluable, as is knowing the questions to ask and when, but be aware that the goalposts may move. Things Mum was adamant about before labour may now feel irrelevant or irritating to her. She could not have predicted everything so if she says the back massage is driving her insane, stop and try something else. If she is now begging for an epidural, check she really wants to go against the birth plan and then support her decision.

How incapacitated is she going to be?

Returning from surgery she may look tired and wan and may be rather groggy and nauseous, especially if she has had a general anaesthetic. This can be rather distressing if you are not prepared for it. Depending on the caesarean circumstances and her reaction to surgery, her level of incapacity in the first 24 hours can be quite a shock. Some mums really cannot get out of bed and when they do hunch over and shuffle to protect the incision. You may find it easier to care for your baby than she in the first few hours as her mobility is slowed by surgery. This phase, if experienced at all, should last no more than a day or two – unless she has been very ill in addition to the surgery.

Help! What on earth do we do now?

Even if one of you has been around babies or young children for any length of time, it can feel quite different when you are responsible for one of your own. Though you will both learn quickly how to hold, comfort and care for her don't be surprised if both of you have moments of self-doubt when you realise you don't know all the answers. Get to know your baby by spending time with her, both in her good moments as well pacing the floor with her at 2 am. Playing an active role both

> **Don't panic**
>
> "It's lying in its crib, staring up at you and thinking, *'You are a bit of an arse, aren't you?'* No it's not. That's just your imagination. Your brand new baby is capable of few thoughts more than *I'm hungry, I'm tired...*" Marcus Berkmann, writer and father[164]

before and after she is born means you are more likely to develop a direct relationship with her and this way you are not waiting to learn everything second-hand. Remember too that at this stage her yells are not manipulative beyond the fact she is hungry, uncomfortable or lonely. The problem of course is working out which one it is.

Will we get through this?

Assuming you are both birth partner and Mum's lover you will probably have concerns about your relationship changing and if it is any help she probably does too. Sometimes feelings can sneak up on you. Minor relationship issues can feel major when everyone lacks time and energy. However, forewarned is forearmed and it helps to talk about how things are changing. It may be helpful to talk to other parents to gain a little perspective before tackling issues head on (see Other resources).

When will we change back?

All the physical and emotional changes you have witnessed and experienced will probably change again after the birth. While much of your old selves will return, you cannot be *exactly* the same.

You may both remain focused on baby related things for quite some time – the primary carer particularly. Your baby demands a lot of time and energy and through necessity will come first. You may not be aware of just how different you both are and even if you are, you may be too exhausted to do anything about it.

In the early days *baby blues* are likely to affect her differently on a minute by minute basis – crying about nothing you can work out one minute and believing she is the world's worst mother the next.

As *baby blues* disappear the reality of daily life may continue to be a shock. Both of you may find that energy levels remain low and moods continue to seesaw. Be proactive. Before difficulties become ingrained talk

> **Recognise pregnancy phases**
>
> "If the physiological upheavals do not get her, the emotional ones will. In the second trimester, during the *glow* or *bloom*, she will be full of energy...but for now all she will want to do is lie on the sofa and eat biscuits." Marcus Berkmann, writer and father[165]

about them and together work out ways to have time together without your baby. Perhaps get a babysitter even if it is only for an hour in the beginning. Getting out of the house and feeling *a bit like the old days* may do you both the world of good. While you may make a pact not to talk about the baby on these occasions, do not be surprised if you do.

Hopefully things should improve as routines develop and you both start to feel a bit more in control. If you find that one of you does not start to improve it is important you recognise this, more help may be needed (see Appendix D).

When can we have sex?

A caesarean does not mean your sex life will be unaffected by a birth. An unplanned caesarean means Mum has probably laboured for some time and may be very uncomfortable for days or weeks afterwards. Even if she did not labour she may not feel like sex any more than after a vaginal birth. There are many reasons for this:

> **Contraception**
>
> Always take contraception seriously. It is a myth that breastfeeding or the absence of her period prevents a new pregnancy.

- She will bleed quite heavily vaginally for days or weeks after the birth and may feel uncomfortable with intimacy

- Her insides may feel battered or out of place from pregnancy and the caesarean and fear of pain may put her off even trying

- The incision may not have healed and she might be worried about exertion causing it to give way (she may worry about this even if it has healed)

- Exhaustion alone will put off some women

- She may feel overweight or less attractive. She will still look 7 months pregnant for several weeks after and some might feel unhappy about being seen naked

- She is likely to be emotionally drained due to all the time and energy she is directing toward the baby

- She may feel apprehensive about how she has changed *down below* and what you might think

- Her breasts may be painful and breastfeeding reduces sex drive in many mums in any case

- It may just feel too soon for no reason she can explain

Knowing when it is all right to resume sex is difficult. The official line is *not before the 6 week check*. At this time the doctor will examine Mum to confirm that bleeding has stopped, her incision has healed and there are no signs of infection or significant on-going discomfort. In theory if she gets a clean bill of health you are both *good to go*. In reality some couples feel ready before this and for others it may not happen for several months. It is important to talk about the reasons. While you may not be able to relate to them, they will feel very real to her. Try not to feel your interest is unreasonable, but the way you approach the discussion is important. You do not want her to feel you are trying to push her into something she is not ready for as it may cause her to withdraw from you completely.

Sex is important in relationships and you may have to encourage her to remember that you are still a couple who need intimacy, despite your baby's demands. This is a very difficult conversation and one that can quickly become highly emotionally charged on both sides, so approach with caution and perhaps talk about this possibility before your baby arrives.

Initially, caressing, massage and foreplay may feel more appropriate than penetrative sex. When you do have sex for the first time be prepared for it to be different. Physical changes and ongoing discomfort may mean she needs different positions. A particularly good one when recovering from a caesarean is *spoons* (see Figure 9). Positions that require Mum to use her stomach muscles too much or which offer little protection for her abdomen (e.g. *doggy* or *missionary*) may be a while returning to the repertoire. Do not be afraid to use assistance to help things along such as pillows to support her and lubrication (she is more likely to need lubrication if she is breastfeeding).

Be prepared for changes in you too:

- Your own sex drive can take a temporary nosedive

- You may have difficulty getting into and staying in the mood when there is a grizzly baby in the room

- You may be afraid of hurting Mum

- Your own exhaustion may leave you uninterested

With time and patience, energy and enthusiasm should return though the frequency may alter.

My recovery

The position of birth partner has rapidly changed in recent decades. It has gone from being female family or friends to the father of the baby, with many fathers choosing or being expected to be involved in the practicalities of birth. There has been little guidance beyond the practical on how to ready yourself for such a life changing experience. Birth is, for many, very emotional and while many of your reactions are likely to be very positive, some may not be. There is no such thing as a *normal* reaction.

The remainder of this chapter concentrates mainly on recovery from negative emotional reactions as it is in these instances that your health, your bond with your baby and your relationship with Mum and siblings can be most affected. Emotional responses are very complex and personal so if need be seek personalised support from skilled practitioners.

How might I feel?

The arrival of your baby can raise many emotions, some more obvious than others. Many will be connected to the birth itself, others more to do with your past or your relationship with Mum. Hormones play a part in this for you as well as Mum. Pheromones produced by your baby can reduce your testosterone levels within minutes of her birth, chemically switching on *parent mode*. Even the prospect of parenthood can start hormonal changes well before her birth.[167] So while we often hear talk of Mum's hormones preparing her for birth, influencing her behaviour and mood, so too can yours.

> **Think positively**
>
> Research looking at fathers reactions to birth found that "the vast majority (93%) are positive about it, even if they have also been frightened or upset." Adrienne Burgess, Head of research at the Fatherhood Institute[166]

Many of the feelings that you will experience during this time are very positive. Strong bonds are formed and wonderful memories created. There will be times however when you feel less positive and in addition to the excitement and euphoria of birth, awe and wonder at the miracle of nature, you may also feel several of the following:

- Ambivalence/disconnection during the pregnancy

- Self-doubt and fear of incompetence when caring for your baby

- Worry about the changes that are coming

- Guilt that you were not able to prevent an unwanted caesarean or alleviate labour pain

- Horror at the physical trauma you witnessed

- Worry that you will not be able to comfort your baby

Following a caesarean your reactions may be influenced in particular by the circumstances leading up to it, the reasons for it, your involvement in it or the strength of your preference (and Mum's) for a specific type of birth. In addition to these you may have more general concerns about finances, work commitments and exhaustion.

All of the above are *normal* and the positive often outweighs the negative, but it is partly in working through all these together that you become a family.

> **Emotional upheaval**
>
> It is a myth that you will not hear your baby crying at night. You are likely to be as disturbed and likely to find your child's crying as measurably stressful as Mum does (increasing your heart rate, skin moisture etc.).[168]

What can I do to help myself?

This section deals primarily with your emotional recovery following a caesarean though many of the ideas apply to the arrival of any baby regardless of how she was born.

Before birth

Take an active role in the pregnancy, attend antenatal appointments and classes and learn about birth, working together to develop the birth plan. By doing so there will be fewer surprises and you will have a better idea of what questions to ask and of whom as you go through each stage.

After birth

Difficult emotions connected with the birth are not unusual. The following list describes the common themes with ways to tackle them. What works for one person will not necessarily work for another so ignore those things that do not feel right for you.

> **Manage expectations**
>
> "Recognising that a C-section is a possibility in any pregnancy and understanding the possible reasons for it may make a woman feel less traumatised emotionally if her delivery suddenly becomes a surgical event, even if the decision for surgical birth is made very rapidly, to save a life or lives." Dr Michele Moore, Physician in Preventative Care and Women's Health [169] et al

- **Lack of control** – Being unable to alleviate pain or change Mum's situation can leave some birth partners feeling powerless and distressed. Some feel they have somehow failed Mum. You may benefit from talking through your side of the experience[170] so take part in the *debrief* (see Chapter 6). Understanding why things happened the way they did may help you and allay some of the guilt. Being stoical is not going to make the feelings go away

> *A dad commenting on a late decision caesarean for a breach baby said "What was so great was that I was the first to bath her, I changed her first nappy with a bit of help from the midwife. I feel really lucky that I did not have to go through the hours of stress and screaming [referring to labour] that I've heard about from friends." Duncan (27)*

- **Self-doubt** – It is not un-common to feel less able to look after your baby than Mum. The more involved you are the more confident you will become as you learn about your baby and begin to recognise her little foibles. Try not to worry about the mistakes you make, everyone does so at one time or another. Mum will make plenty too

- **Home alone** – The first couple of nights after a caesarean birth you are likely to be at home without Mum or your baby. This can feel like a major anticlimax (even if you do have other siblings to care for) and some partners feel distressed by the separation as well as exhausted. You may want company or prefer to be on your own so think carefully before having all the relatives over to celebrate. If they are coming from a distance, consider putting them up with friends so you have periods of time to yourself if that is what you need. Take care of yourself, eat properly and rest – this is the calm before the storm. Once Mum and baby come home, sleepless nights and the anxieties associated with new routines will be upon you

- **Detached** – The baby tends to take centre stage and while understandable, it can leave you rather isolated. Those around you are less likely to be looking out for you, instead expecting you to be the support for everyone else. Your own *stiff upper lip* may of course be disguising the strength of your feelings but do not let it continue too long, talk to Mum and try to work out a new path

- **Competitive exhaustion** – Mum has a really obvious drag on her health, humour, energy levels, mood etc. and it is relatively easy for her and others to forget that a similar experience is happening to you too. This can result in the destructive condition of *competitive exhaustion*. Here couples get locked in a spiral of whose day is worse, who is more tired, who has the worst deal. For totally different reasons you are both facing incredibly difficult times and it is very easy for resentment and blame to set in, putting considerable strain on your relationship. The illustration below shows a classic example where Mum is the primary carer on maternity leave and the partner is the primary breadwinner.

Partner is working a full day then coming home to be with the family, taking on additional activities, dealing with a maelstrom of emotions from Mum, experiencing the whole gamut of challenges from the baby, all while being utterly sleep deprived.	**Mum** feels she has sacrificed her identity, is stifled by mind-numbing monotony with little adult conversation and while she may remember to nap when baby sleeps, she has something literally sucking the energy out of her 10 times a day, all while extremely sleep deprived.

This is a difficult situation for both parties but for quite different reasons. Recognising what is happening and talking about it can start to address the issue, but it is only in truly believing the roles are vastly different and have extreme and unique pressures of their own, that you can hope to remove this barrier to emotional recovery. Work out what is reasonable for each of you to be doing. Be honest about what you need and find a middle ground. If you need 10 minutes to *change hats* when you walk through the door at the end of a working day, say so, as long as you can accept that sometimes her day will have been so stressful the only way she has made it to your *home time* is by counting the minutes until she could literally hand the baby over to you

- **Depression** – The changes in these early days are massive. A day at work may feel like a welcome break by comparison. Unfortunately when you come home to recharge this is likely to be the last thing you get a chance to do. These changes coupled with exhaustion and some or all of the above leave you susceptible to depression, and you are more likely to become depressed if Mum is depressed.[171] Birth partners (male or female) can suffer from a form of postnatal depression. This condition is little known and certainly poorly understood so it is important you recognise

> **Negative reactions to the birth event**
>
> "Fathers can feel let down by the birth experience – feeling distressed at having been in a situation where, even after antenatal classes, they didn't really know how or where to help. Some feel their time in hospital overly controlled, restricting rather than supporting their bond with their baby, stating they would prefer to let the bond with their child unfold over time."
> Penny Christensen, Birth Trauma Canada

what is happening and seek support from online groups and counselling services if need be (see Appendix D)

Paternal postnatal depression

Paternal postnatal depression (PPnD), also known as Male Postnatal Depression is not well-known, yet a Danish study suggests that depression rates in fathers of new babies are double the national average for men in the same age group.[172] If undiagnosed, PPnD can make life difficult for you and those around you and can lead to the break up of relationships because the resulting behaviours are so difficult to cope with[173] (see Appendix D).

Treatment for PPnD is essential – it is unlikely to go away on its own. Many men do not voice their negative feelings, believing they are protecting Mum but this can make the situation a lot worse. It is important that you seek help, one-to-one counselling and local support groups can offer an opportunity to voice fears and feelings

> **Possible side effect of PnD**
>
> If left untreated PnD in either partner is thought to account for the increased rate of relationship breakdown within the first year of a child arriving.[174]

in a safe environment (see Other resources). Simply hiding your difficulties hinders your own recovery. Getting together face-to-face or online with other partners in similar situations can help you feel less alone and provide you with a support network to lean on if need be. Talk to your doctor, they may have information about local support services and counsellors or if you prefer go on-line (see Other resources). Try to make time for yourself and keep a hobby going so there is still some space for you.

The caesarean procedure

Knowing what is involved in a caesarean can make a big difference to how you feel facing the experience. For some women the more they know, the worse they feel; for others, the more information they have the better. Certainly the more you know, the more you can influence your experience and the more influence you have, the more personal and positive your caesarean birth is likely to feel.

It is equally important you understand the full implications of a vaginal birth (see Appendix C). It can involve just as much poking and prodding, medical intervention and drugs as a caesarean just in different areas of the body. Recovery afterwards can present just as many surprises too. This can come as quite a shock to many women when antenatal education has not presented the complete picture.

What will happen?

The following description is of a planned caesarean with the differences for unplanned caesareans highlighted at the end of the chapter.

In the days leading up to the caesarean

A blood test

Seven days prior to the planned date a blood test is conducted to check your haemoglobin levels. It also confirms your blood group in case a transfusion is necessary.

A tablet to stop your stomach making acid

Taken the night before, this helps reduce acid and nausea when used in conjunction with another tablet on the day of surgery.

No food

Your last meal is the night before surgery. You will not eat again until afterwards, though water is OK up to two hours before surgery.

Hospital arrival time

The time you are given is typically quite specific and probably several hours before surgery. Stick to this as hospital schedules can be tight. However other women's emergency caesareans will be prioritised over your planned caesarean so surgery time may alter.

On arrival at hospital

Identity bracelet

A bracelet will be supplied by the hospital with your name and a code, it will remain on your wrist for the duration of your stay.

Antacid

Your second acid suppressant is due.

Change into your gown

The hospital will supply a gown, it opens at the back! Turn it round if you are hoping to breastfeed in theatre.

Put on knee length surgical stockings

These are far from sexy but important in protecting against blood clots. Some hospitals use inflatable shoes during surgery instead or inject a blood-thinning agent (heparin). It is important that your hospital offers you one of these options.

Shaving

If you have not shaved your pubic area in advance, most hospitals will do this for you. Do not expect anything high tech, you will probably be standing in a nearby toilet cubicle with a nurse, a disposable razor and no shaving cream. If you want to do this yourself it is not necessary to shave the whole area, just that close to the bikini line.

Remove jewellery

You can keep one special ring if it is covered in tape. You will have to remove dentures and all nail varnish – usually fingers and toes (the natural colour of your nails is used by the anaesthetist to detect early changes in your oxygen levels).

Sign a consent form

You may have signed this already at your last appointment. This confirms you have been fully informed about the procedure and its risks. It will ask you to understand these risks, such as infection, excessive bleeding, damage to bladder/bowel, clot formation and death, are possible with surgery. This all looks very scary and even when you have done lots of research it can cause moments of doubt. [More info.xii]

Before surgery begins

Gowning up

Your birth partner will be taken away for a moment to gown up. He may not rejoin you until you are fully prepared for surgery. Some hospitals ask the birth partner to wait outside until epidurals and IVs have been inserted.

People present

In theatre there will be a number of people and lots of technology. This can be daunting but it is all there to make your birth go smoothly. People likely to be present are:

- Your birth partner
- A surgeon and their assistant
- An anaesthetist and their assistant
- A midwife (one for each baby if it is a multiple birth)
- A paediatrician (one for each baby and a resuscitation team if it is known in advance that your baby is experiencing difficulties)
- A theatre nurse (in charge of instruments)
- Additional nurses (one for the anaesthetist and one runner – fetching things as needed)
- Students may be observing

Once in theatre

Anaesthetics

You will be prepared for surgery and talked through each step:

- An IV (intravenous tube) will be inserted into the back of your hand to deliver extra drugs and fluids as needed
- Whilst sitting or side-lying in a curved position, a small area of your back will be numbed before the epidural/spinal is given (see Figure 11). If you are already in labour the tube is inserted between contractions. You will feel pressure on your spine and maybe a slight tingling sensation – it should not be painful

---

xii www.rcog.org.uk search for Consent Advice no. 7 Caesarean Birth

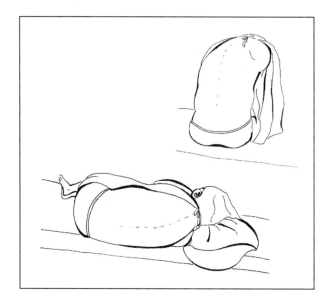

Figure 11 – Epidural positions

- Testing the anaesthetic follows strict protocols to ensure a full block is achieved. It may be a cold spray or touch, first on your arm so you have something to compare with then sprayed in stages up your abdomen and chest asking you to state when you can start to feel the cold/touch sensation. You should only be able to feel it when it reaches your chest. Once complete, additional checks may be carried out e.g. pinching the incision site using a clamp. This may feel like dull pressure but certainly not pain

- Your anaesthetist will remain with you throughout surgery

- A general anaesthetic procedure differs somewhat. In theatre a tube will be inserted into the back of your hand to provide drugs to start and maintain the anaesthetic. It is also used to supply additional drugs (antibiotics) to fight infection, reduce nausea and keep you hydrated. Occasionally gas is used to put you to sleep *before* the anaesthetic. Once asleep a mask or tube will help you breathe properly and is only removed when you are fully awake. When you come round you will be monitored until you are fully awake [More info.[xiii]]

[xiii] www.oaa.anaes.ac.uk search for Your anaesthetic for caesarean section

Settling down

Once fully prepared you will be helped to lie on your back, slightly tilted to the side, with your birth partner seated next to your head. If they have not been with you up to now, this is typically when they are brought into theatre.

There are stories of women having their hands restrained during surgery. If you are awake there is absolutely no reason for this – it is certainly not necessary to counteract the slight tilt of the table. If you are concerned that this may happen, discuss this beforehand.

Catheter

A catheter is inserted *after* the anaesthetic has taken effect to empty your bladder. Ideally it should remain in place for no more than 12 hours.[175] Its removal is usually painless and early removal reduces the likelihood of infection.

The screen

A screen will be raised over your chest to shield your view of surgery and help keep the surgical area sterile. Your gown will be raised up to your chest. Check it is not trapped if you want to have immediate skin-to-skin contact or to breastfeed during surgery.

Iodine

This is sometimes used as an antiseptic to sterilise the incision site. It can leave a pale brown stain in your belly button for a couple weeks but will disappear naturally.

By now the anaesthetic should have taken effect. If labour has started you may feel mild contractions as it does so. It can feel strange but more like period pain than a contraction and sensation quickly subsides.

During surgery

In a straightforward, planned caesarean the whole procedure should take 30-45 minutes, with your baby being delivered in the first 5-10 minutes. The remaining time is cleaning and closing. The set-up time prior to this may have taken as much as an hour.

The anaesthetist and surgeon are usually talking to you explaining what is happening, and the atmosphere is generally very relaxed and informal. For some women the tone can feel like inappropriate banter while others find it puts them at ease. You can ask questions at any time. Many of the sensations can be explained and managed. In particular, if you feel breathless, say so. When they calculate the amount of anaesthetic it is based on several factors and everyone reacts slightly differently. They would rather give you too much than too little so on occasions the block can mean you no longer feel yourself breathing, though you are. If you are one of the rare few whose anaesthetic begins to wear off during surgery, let your anaesthetist know immediately. The surgeon can pause while an anaesthetic top-up improves your situation.

Your birth partner generally remains with you until asked to go to one side with your baby while she is checked.

The incision

A skin is cut in a slight curve along the bikini line, usually for a distance of about 20cm (see Figure 12). The abdominal muscles are separated. The bladder is pushed down or moved to one side to allow a small cut in the peritoneum (the membrane that lines the abdominal cavity). Finally a small horizontal cut is made in the wall of the uterus – occasionally a vertical T or J shape incision may be necessary (see Appendix C).

After the initial incisions are made the openings are sometimes extended *bluntly* i.e. torn, using a finger to part muscles.

Occasionally the external incision will be vertical but this is rare and is dictated by the position of your baby and the speed with which she needs to be delivered (see Figure 13). The internal scar is not necessarily the same as the external one, so check which you have had if you are planning further pregnancies.

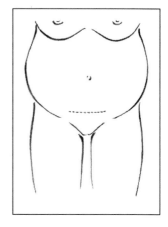

Figure 12 – Horizontal incision

Fluid removal

Once the incisions have all been made, the fluid that cushioned your baby (amniotic fluid) is suctioned away (a rather loud slurping sound).

Delivery

This feels rather like intense tugging or rummaging. There should not be any sharp pain. Some women experience breathlessness during the actual moment of birth because it maybe necessary to push your baby out. In such cases someone will apply pressure behind your baby (on your upper abdomen) restricting (but not stopping) your breathing momentarily.

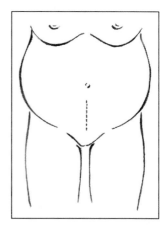

Figure 13 – Vertical incision

New developments referred to as the *natural caesarean* allow your baby to remain partially delivered for some minutes (see Chapter 1). This gives her chance to experience lung compression and acclimatise to her surroundings before she is lifted from you.

The cord

The cord is cut and your baby lifted so you can see her before she is taken to be checked (or straight to you if this has been agreed). You may wish to discuss delaying the cutting of the cord (see Chapter 5).

Antibiotics

These are administered through the IV after the cord has been clamped. This is given as a precaution, to reduce the possibility of infection.

Baby checks

Your baby is weighed and measured and an APGAR score (on a range of 1-10) assesses her breathing, heart rate, muscle tone, colour and reflexes. She will be given a score at 1 minute after birth and again at 5 minutes.

Feeding/cuddling

Your baby is returned to you and your birth partner can help hold her on your upper chest (it feels like she is tucked under your chin). You can try feeding if you wish. Alternatively your birth partner can hold her skin-to-skin or wrapped so that you can both touch and see her. The anaesthetist and surgeon will generally stop their commentary at this point so you can concentrate on your baby – say if you want them to continue.

Extending the incision
Torn tissue heals better than when cut. When muscle is cut, it is done so *along* the muscle so that the fibres can, on the whole, remain intact. On rare occasions a vertical incision may be required. In such cases muscles will need to be cut and recovery will take longer.

Closure

This can take 45 minutes, longer if you have had previous caesareans and there is more scar tissue to accommodate. You will be given a drug to start uterus contraction and stem bleeding. A suction tube removes remaining fluid. The incision is closed layer by layer. Dissolvable stitches are used internally and often externally too. Check whether dissolvable ones will be used externally and find out

Longer surgery time
If there are adhesions from previous surgery it may be more than 10 minutes before your baby is delivered. This does not mean there is anything wrong just that the surgeon is proceeding more slowly to avoid additional damage to you.

why if not. Non-dissolvable stitches or metal stapes are removed usually within 5 days.

A bandage then covers the incision, pressure bandages are sometimes used, these extend across your whole abdomen and are fantastic for making you feel everything is being held in place.

After surgery

Recovery room

You will be taken, along with your birth partner and baby, to a recovery room for between 30 minutes and 4 hours depending on your condition. You will remain connected to a number of monitors, but your upper body is raised, making it easier to hold, see and feed your baby. Here a midwife or nurse will monitor you before your release onto the postnatal ward.

Pain relief

The type offered varies. You will be given some pain relief before leaving theatre (through the IV or a suppository), following which you will be given one of the following:

- Tablet regime

- PCA (Patient Controlled Anaesthetic) regime

- Long-acting epidural or spinal

- Injection

Note – Some types of pain relief have a short intense duration while others are milder but longer lasting. Confirm the type you are on so you know what to expect. It is important pain medication is given according to a strict schedule as even a half hour delay can result in unnecessary pain. Postnatal wards are very busy so watch your times and request your medication if need be. Once a routine is broken it is difficult to get the pain totally back under control. "It is easier to keep pain away than treat it." (Dr Bryan Beattie, Consultant in Fetal Medicine[176])

Checks

Your condition is checked every half hour for the first 2 hours: respiratory rate, heart rate, blood pressure, pain level. Checks become less frequent as your condition improves, at which point staff concentrate on signs of infection.

Removal of equipment

The IV may remain for several hours, providing fluids to rehydrate you. Your catheter will remain until you can walk to the toilet unless there has been damage to the bladder during surgery, in which case it may remain for a week or more. Occasionally a drain at the incision site collects blood that otherwise might pool under the scar, but it is usually removed within 2 days.

Your stay

Typically you will be walking within 12 hours of surgery and expected to stay in hospital for at least 48 hours. This can be longer (3-4 days) if you or your baby are taking longer to recover.

Hospital support

Professional support can be very useful for first time mums trying to get to grips with baby care and breastfeeding. Staff are there to help and can be a wonderful resource, though at busy times they might not be able to help straightaway. Some can be quite opinionated about what you should and should not be doing, particularly in relation to breastfeeding, and advice can be contradictory. Listen but do *not* allow yourself to be bullied into something you do not feel ready or able to do.

Baby checks

After the initial checks (see above) there will be others within 48 hours, these include a complete physical check-up, observation of feeding, nappy condition, hearing and light sensitivity etc. [More info. [xiv]]

A planned caesarean after labour begins

There are a few differences to the procedure above if you have already gone into *normal* labour i.e. there are no complications and your baby has simply decided it is time to arrive. This is *not* a true emergency so most elements of the procedure should remain the same and any specific requests you made in your birth plan should still stand.

- The speed with which everything happens may be quicker

- You may not have taken your first acid suppressant – a liquid antacid will be given instead. It is not quite as effective so you may feel some nausea

- The insertion of needles will be timed to take account of contractions

- The surgeon will be operating through contracting muscle, slightly increasing the possibility of nicks to other organs in the vicinity and to your baby

---

[xiv] www.babycentre.co.uk search for Newborn baby tests and checks

- You may labour for longer than you would like, while staff and facilities become available

- If you have laboured for a significant period you are likely to feel quite bruised and tired afterwards

An unplanned caesarean

An unplanned caesarean is one of two types: emergency or critical (see Chapter 1). In either case the unplanned nature means that the experience will at times feel quite different to that of a planned caesarean.

One of the most significant differences is the type of emotional response you may have. Feelings linked with lack of control,[177] fear of surgery, loss of privacy or fear of the unknown can all suddenly come into play, even for women who have investigated this possibility. All this is in addition to the worry associated with the medical emergency itself.

An emergency caesarean

- You may be asked to sign a consent form before surgery, although many maternity units do not require this as consent given by someone in a hurry and in pain is not legally valid in any case. This could be a little daunting as you may not have had time to take it in or ask as many questions as you would like, though the reasons for the caesarean and how it will be done should still be briefly explained to you prior to surgery

- You will be moved from your labour room to theatre with more people present

- Everything happens quicker, leaving less time for explanations

- Your anaesthesia will typically be regional so that you can still be awake for your birth

- You will not have taken your first acid suppressant – a liquid antacid will be administered that is not quite as effective so you may feel some nausea

- If you are in labour the insertion of needles will be timed to take account of contractions

- The decision to have a caesarean has been taken, but you may have to wait until staff and facilities become available

- On delivery your baby will be checked (see – this chapter) and sometimes taken to the SCU for further assistance

- If you have laboured first you are likely to feel quite bruised and tired afterwards

A critical caesarean

- Time permitting you may be asked to sign the consent form. You will not have time to ask questions

- Ideally a regional anaesthetic is used but in some cases a general is required to put you to sleep quickly so your baby can be delivered as soon as possible

- You may not have time for the acid suppressant and may feel rather sick for a time

- You may not be awake as your baby is born but if all is well your birth partner will be able to look after her until you come round

- Your birth partner will not be with you if a general anaesthetic is necessary

- There is a greater risk of surgical injury to you and your baby, due to the speed of delivery

- On delivery your baby will be checked (see – this chapter) and may be taken to the SCU

- You and your baby are likely to feel drowsy after a general anaesthetic

- If you have laboured first you are likely to feel quite bruised and tired afterwards

Why do caesareans happen?

Caesareans are costly and associated with a higher risk of negative outcomes than straightforward vaginal births. However not all pregnancies are straightforward and a caesarean may be recommended or be required. The following classifications[178] are often used to categorise your situation:

- There is an immediate threat to your or your baby's life (level 1)

- You or your baby are compromised but it is not immediately life-threatening (level 2)

- Neither you nor your baby are compromised but would benefit from early delivery (level 3)

- Delivery is timed to suit you or staff availability (level 4)

Some reasons are clear cut, others less so. Understanding the distinctions can make all the difference to your ability to negotiate before or during your birth. Some situations may leave you with weeks/days to prepare, others require immediate surgery or in others it may be that a vaginal birth is still possible.

Doctor's recommendation

A doctor's recommendation is sometimes just that – a recommendation – vaginal birth could still be a possibility. In other situations it is really the only option. Your understanding of *suggested* versus *required* can directly determine the course of your birth. For example, breech does not automatically mean a caesarean, though practitioners usually recommend it if they have been unable to turn your baby into a head down position. A combination of factors is leading some practitioners to err on the side of caution and offer caesareans when a vaginal birth may still be possible.

When is a caesarean considered the best or only option?

In some situations a caesarean can offer significant benefits over an attempted vaginal birth. The following are situations where a caesarean is typically considered the best or only option.

Prior to labour

Prior to labour certain conditions occur during pregnancy, or are part of your medical history which indicate a caesarean is the best way to deliver your baby.

High order multiple births i.e. 3 or more babies

Due to the higher risks associated with multiple births (for each baby), practitioners often recommend caesareans. Vaginal birth is still possible but generally only considered if your midwife is very experienced with multiple births. Over 92% of UK triplets are born by caesarean.[179] Take a look at your hospital's statistics to understand their preference and experience. If they routinely recommend caesareans this will reduce their experience with vaginal, high order multiple birth deliveries and reduce your chances of gaining agreement to attempt it.

Transverse position

Babies lying across your abdomen rather than head or bottom down are difficult to turn and unless she turns you will require a caesarean.

Placenta praevia

A placenta implanted low in the wall of your uterus may partially or entirely block your baby's exit. Significant cervical blockage (identified via ultrasound) requires a caesarean due to the likelihood of severe bleeding as the cervix dilates during labour. Have a scan around week 36 as the placenta can *move* during pregnancy to the extent that you may be able to give birth vaginally. This condition occurs in approximately 5 in 1,000[180] of US pregnancies, the likelihood increasing with the number of caesareans you have (see Appendix C). [More info.[xv]]

Placental accrete

The placenta grows deeply into the muscle of the uterus wall. Although it can happen in any pregnancy the likelihood increases after previous uterine surgery (this includes caesareans, some types of surgery for fibroids and where there is infection following uterine evacuation of pregnancy) and when there is a placenta praevia.[181] It is difficult to diagnose and the main problem arises when the placenta fails to separate normally or fully. Since it is very deeply embedded significant bleeding can occur requiring surgery to stem the bleeding and detach the placenta. In very rare severe cases a hysterectomy may be necessary due to persistent life threatening bleeding (see Appendix 10).

[xv] www.rcog.org.uk search for A low-lying placenta after 20 weeks

Placental abruption

The oxygen supply to your baby is interrupted as the placenta prematurely separates from the uterus. This occurs in approximately 1 in 100 births and has been associated with high blood pressure. If blood loss and separation is significant it will be necessary to deliver your baby immediately via caesarean – or forceps if you are already in the second stage of labour.

Scar rupture

Rarely an old caesarean scar will re-open. This will usually lead to a caesarean (see Chapter 4 & Appendix C).

Pre-eclampsia

This condition is characterised by high blood pressure, water retention, protein in the urine, abdominal pain and light sensitivity. This condition is brought on by pregnancy, and can only be resolved by your baby being delivered. Pre-eclampsia occurs in approx 2-3 in 100 births.[182][183] In mild cases your condition can be managed and you may go on to deliver vaginally. If treatment is not working or you progress to eclampsia (1 in 2,000 pregnancies) then it will be necessary to have a caesarean. [More info.[xvi]]

HELLP

A group of symptoms: Haemolysis, Elevated Liver enzymes and Low Platelet count (the same as pre-eclampsia but with additional evidence of liver damage and abnormal blood clotting). Various approaches can be taken to manage the condition. If these are not working immediate delivery via caesarean will be necessary.

Maternal conditions

Some conditions suggest you may not be able to cope with a protracted vaginal birth e.g. high blood pressure, lung or heart disease, previous vaginal surgery (e.g. a prolapse repair) or diabetes (if not under control), though even then if labour starts spontaneously and progresses well you may be able to give birth vaginally. In addition, previous injuries involving the pelvis may mean that it is too misshapen to allow your baby to safely pass through and a caesarean will be required.

Fetal illness, abnormality or poor growth

Significant fetal complications can mean your baby may not survive a protracted vaginal birth and a caesarean may be safer. Such complications might be: heart conditions, poor growth or water on the brain causing an enlarged head (hydrocephalus).

[xvi] www.rcog.org.uk search for Pre-eclampsia-what you need to know

HIV or genital herpes outbreak

You can pass infectious diseases to your baby via blood, vaginal fluids or breast milk. Transmission *may* be managed more effectively with a caesarean.[184] So while a caesarean does not benefit you, it may benefit your baby. However, in the UK practitioners are tending to recommend, for women with an undetectable viral load (where treatment has already proven effective), that a caesarean is optional. In the case of genital herpes, if the outbreak is prior to your third trimester you should produce antibodies that will be passed to your baby during pregnancy enabling you to safely give birth vaginally. It is only when a *confirmed first* outbreak occurs in the third trimester or within 6 weeks of your due date that a planned caesarean is recommended. If you continue to pursue a vaginal birth in this situation there are significant risks of neonatal herpes. It is very important that the membranes are not ruptured and other invasive procedures such as fetal scalp electrodes need to be avoided.[185]

During labour

Unplanned caesareans occur when one of the conditions above goes undetected. In addition to these there are other conditions which may only occur or become obvious during labour. If the following situations arise you are more likely to have a caesarean.

Large baby

Sometimes a baby's head is too big to pass through your pelvis. This is known as cephalopelvic disproportion and will require a caesarean. A large head in a previous pregnancy does not necessarily mean the same this time (unless you have diabetes). It is quite difficult to accurately assess the size of your baby near to term and therefore a large baby may only become obvious as your labour progresses. Equally the inaccuracies of ultrasound means that often babies thought to be large antenatally turn out to be average size, so take this into account when debating the need for a caesarean for this reason prior to labour.

Heavy bleeding

When heavy bleeding cannot be controlled a caesarean may be required to deliver your baby quickly so that the cause of the bleeding can also be treated.

Umbilical cord compression

Cord compression can sometimes be managed so you can continue to labour, but not in all cases. Your specific situation and the extent to which your baby is coping will dictate the urgency of the situation.

Cord prolapse

If the umbilical cord falls through into the vagina ahead of your baby the cord can be compressed causing fetal distress due to oxygen starvation. Cord prolapse occurs in 1 in 200 births[186] and in most cases requires immediate caesarean unless you can deliver within the next few minutes.

Fetal distress

This becomes evident through a drop or irregularity in your baby's heart rate or her passing meconium (baby poo). However, *normal* fluctuations in heart rates can occur naturally during birth and an experienced midwife will know the difference. Time permitting, fetal blood sampling can check whether a baby is critically short of oxygen and if so, a caesarean or assisted vaginal delivery (in the 2nd stage of labour) will be carried out.

Exhaustion

A lengthy labour with little progress can cause exhaustion to the extent you are no longer able to labour effectively and a caesarean may be recommended.

When is a caesarean a possibility but not critical?

In the following situations you are likely to be offered a caesarean.

Breech position

Your baby is lying bottom down – 2-3 in 100 single babies are breech at term[187] (see Figure 14). With an experienced practitioner and no other complications you can try a vaginal birth. However find out the approximate size of your baby and the position of her head. These factors affect your chances. [More info.xvii] Over 50% of vaginal attempts are successful, but research indicates planned caesareans before labour have better outcomes for the baby as so many breech vaginal deliveries involve instrumental intervention.[188] Make sure you understand the risks (e.g. cord prolapse, instrumental intervention or an unplanned caesarean), and be very clear about the experience of your midwife. As the number of vaginal breech deliveries decreases some midwives

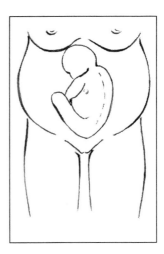

Figure 14 – Breech position

---

are not gaining sufficient experience to confidently deliver a breech baby. [More info.[xviii]]

Other awkward positions

An asynclitic position, where your baby's head is tilted so it is not in line with the birth canal can cause a protracted labour. Babies lying this way may correct their position naturally as labour progresses, but where they do not you will need a caesarean.

Late baby

Induction starts to be offered from week 41 and if you go over 42 weeks many practitioners strongly advise induction because babies can become too big to deliver vaginally. Fewer fetal deaths occur in pregnancies where intervention takes place around week 41 but the overall risk is very small even at 42 weeks.[189] Induction has been connected with an increased likelihood of a caesarean outcome.[190]

Previous caesarean

On average 25% of all caesareans are performed following a previous caesarean.[191] Some practitioners offer a repeat caesarean due to concerns about scar rupture during labour (see Appendix C) and in some places you may find you have difficulty gaining agreement for a VBAC. The US and UK have committed to a target of just under 40% VBACs.[192] Assuming there are no other obvious issues you should be able to try vaginal birth if you wish (see Chapter 4).

Multiple births

In the UK 59% of multiple births are caesareans, of which 37% are planned and 63% unplanned and 92% of triplets are born by caesarean.[193] The premise for many caesarean recommendations is that one or more baby is lying in a difficult position or there are concerns about cord entanglement. Statistics also show that multiple births run a higher risk of low birth weight or premature delivery.[194] With additional risk factors such as an increased risk of death of the second twin[195] and possibilities of emergency situations after the vaginal delivery of the first twin (around 10% of second twins are born via caesarean)[196] it is generally recommended that twins be delivered via caesarean around week 37-8.[197] A study looking at twins born by planned caesarean found the risk of death to be negligible.[198] However, where there are no other complications and your babies are both lying in a good position you may be able to attempt a vaginal birth. As the number of vaginal multiple deliveries decreases some midwives are not gaining

---

[xviii] www.cmaj.ca article by Hannah M search for cmaj Planned elective caesarean section & www.ncbi.nlm.nih.gov article by Hofmery GJ Planned caesarean section for breech delivery

sufficient experience to confidently deliver, so again be very clear about the experience of your midwifery team before making a decision.

Failure to progress (Dystocia)

All sorts of things may cause your labour to slow, stop or go slower than expected: e.g. moving from home to hospital, the position of your baby or conflicting dilation measurements (these are subjective and variation can occur with each new person taking the measurement).[199] These things in isolation do not mean you need a caesarean. Significant delay can, however, cause fetal distress and you should be clear about the level and type of distress before rejecting a caesarean recommendation.

Pre-term labour

In situations where labour begins very early, practitioners may recommend a caesarean if they think your baby is unlikely to cope with the rigors of vaginal birth.

Your age

The older you are the more likely you are to have a caesarean[200] [201] or instrumental delivery.[202] The exact cause is unclear though age related complications[203] (e.g. pre-eclampsia and diabetes)[204] and an increased nervousness (due to your age) on the part of you or your practitioner are thought to play a part.[205] One commentator suggests given the "chances of a spontaneous vaginal delivery decreases with each year [women] delay childbirth"[206] they should be informed of this and perhaps even able to "request an elective caesarean section to avoid the high risk of emergency operative delivery." (Adam Rosenthal, Clinical Research fellow, St Bartholomew's Hospital, London[207]) However another commentator has suggested that the assumption that older mothers are more at risk of complications creates a "fear of complications" increasingly the likelihood of women planning a caesarean. Therefore "each caesarean performed on an older woman, will not only enter statistics that purport to show that older women have more problems giving birth vaginally, but will also become part of the 'culture of childbirth' that instils fear of birth in other pregnant women. Thus fear perpetuates fear." (Jane Weaver, Research Associate, Centre for Family Research, University of Cambridge[208])

Your physical characteristics

The heavier or shorter you are and the higher your BMI the more likely you are to have a caesarean.[209] [210] This is thought to be due to medical complications associated with obese mothers. Conditions such as pre-eclampsia are more common (11% in obese mothers while only 2% in lighter mothers). Obese mothers are more likely to have babies at the extreme ends of birth weight charts and either become stuck and/or show signs of fetal distress requiring a caesarean.[211] Being overweight is connected with a 50% increase in the likelihood of caesarean delivery "more than double for obese women compared with women with normal BMI." (Dr Amudha Pooblan et al[212]) An obese mother also faces longer surgery time and this has been connected with worse outcomes such as incision infection.[213]

Ethnicity

Certain medical conditions typically leading to caesareans are more prevalent in some ethnic groups e.g. diabetes and pre-eclampsia in black women.[214]

Why might some women request a caesarean?

Occasionally women request caesareans (Caesarean Delivery on Maternal Request – CDMR). Media coverage often labels these women *too posh to push* but in actual fact the situation is far more complicated.

Studies[215] have produced wildly differing figures about CDMR rates, anything from 75 in 10,000[216] to 2,800 in 10,000.[217] Such discrepancies in CDMR figures are due to a combination of:

- Variation in data collection methods (different categorisation protocols between practitioners and hospitals)

- Inaccurate record keeping

- Biased study design

Medical records often describe a decision as *maternal request* even if:

- The caesarean was first recommended by the practitioner[218]

- The woman believes that a medical situation implies a caesarean may be preferable[219]

Unfortunately many studies include caesareans carried out following a practitioner's recommendation. In other words, the woman has chosen a caesarean after a specific recommendation from her practitioner because of her circumstances, not just because she wants one.

Some requests appear to involve very specific cultural reasons. The 20% CDMR rate[220] in parts of China is thought to result from a combination of the *precious baby* phenomenon i.e. a *prophylactic* caesarean (one planned to specifically avoid certain outcomes - perhaps because the mother is over 35 or has had difficulty conceiving) and Chinas single child policy which has removed some risks associated with future pregnancies.

In many cases previous birth experience and pregnancy complications appear to account for the maternal requests[221] but the picture is far from clear.

The following are common reasons mothers may give for requesting a caesarean. The extent to which these carry any weight with practitioners may be a matter of hospital policy or personal opinion.

Previous experience

Some women who have already experienced a caesarean (even an unplanned one) would rather go through the same mode of birth again as to them it is a *known quantity*. For others if their previous vaginal birth was traumatic and complicated, they may now be afraid of labour. For these women a planned caesarean feels more acceptable than labour with the chances of an emergency arising which may result in an unplanned caesarean. Requesting a caesarean on such grounds is sometimes referred to as a *prophylactic* caesarean – a proactive choice to avoid certain outcomes.

Fear of childbirth

> **A perspective on caesareans**
>
> A study looking at mothers' decision-making and birth choices found that when needing to consider caesareans many referred to planned caesareans as "a more favourable option than risking labour that might end in an emergency...they perceived [it] as an ordered process of events and, perhaps more significantly, under the control of the professionals." Jane Weaver, Researcher from the Centre for Family Research, University of Cambridge [222] et al [More info.[xix]]

Although childbirth is a natural process, it is unpredictable and, for most, painful. Fear is thought to be a common reason behind CDMR. Its frequency is unclear with reported rates varying significantly,[223] [224] [225] although overall the incidence appears to be rising. It is often given as the primary reason for a request caesarean[226] and is certainly reflected in an increase in the use and preference for pain relief.[227]

The root of the fear may be: throw away comments from practitioners or friends, negative experiences of friends or family members, media images,[228] [229] or concerns about pelvic floor damage – the latter typically reported by practitioners (not mothers).[230] Previous birth trauma[231] and prior abuse account for some requests.[232] It may also be the result of more ambiguous

> *A mum talking about her emergency caesarean said "I had an emergency section after W did not turn from breech and it was all taking too long. The caesarean happened so fast. I've had flashbacks ever since. I am not sure I can go through the whole birth thing again." Meg (31)*

[xix] Login it's worth reading – www.electivecesareans.com search for 'caesarean on maternal request'

thoughts such as: a general fear of pain, dying, medical intervention, fear of mothers own incompetence during delivery, a lack of trust in practitioners[233] or simply fear of the unknown.

The level of fear varies but for some it can become a *morbid dread* and the fear of surgery may actually hold far less significance for the woman than fear of vaginal birth. With this condition some women even choose to remain childless or abort much wanted babies.[234] It is known as tokophobia[235] and can hamper a woman's ability to cope with and progress through her labour and subsequent recovery. Forcing women suffering from tokophobia to labour causes them greater emotional distress than those permitted a caesarean.[236]

Regardless of mode of delivery, approximately 2 in 100 women have such negative reactions to their birth that their symptoms register on the PTSD scale.[237] In the case of unplanned caesareans as many as a third of women may experience "intrusive stress reactions" (Dr Elsa Lena Ryding, Obstetric Consultant[238] et al) (see Chapter 6 & Appendix D). The on-going impact of such reactions can significantly influence a woman's preferences about the way she wants to give birth. Being able to maintain some *feeling* of control over birth has been

> **Tokophobia**
>
> This term describes a severe dread of childbirth. Primary tokophobia pre-dates any pregnancy. Secondary tokophobia occurs following a previous traumatic event during pregnancy or childbirth. In both cases women may be so affected they request caesareans to avoid labour or actively avoid becoming pregnant.

shown to be of fundamental importance to women.[239] "Even if the birth was not natural as planned, women were still pleased with the experience if they felt they had been in control of the decisions made." (Joanne E Lally, Research Fellow at Institute of Health and Society, Newcastle University[240])

Despite numerous studies stating that tokophobia affects a woman's ability to labour effectively[241] and that it can result in poor emotional outcomes, many countries do not formally recognise fear of childbirth as a reason for CDMR.

If you are experiencing a significant level of fear your hospital may recommend counselling. While research indicates that professional support of this sort can reduce the level of fear and increase confidence in *some* women so that they are able to face vaginal birth,[242] [243] for others it will simply not be enough[244] and a caesarean may feel like the only option for them.

> *A mum's reason for requesting a planned caesarean after an unplanned one, "I really wanted to remember this birth. I was totally out of it last time. I managed to hold L in theatre and even feed him there too. It really put to rest the awfulness of my first caesarean." Sarah (37)*

Personal circumstances

The circumstances of your pregnancy may place you in a *higher risk group* (see – this chapter). In some hospitals a caesarean will automatically be recommended, in others it will be down to you to state a preference.

Older women seem more inclined toward CDMR (34+),[245] particularly if pregnancy follows one or more IVF procedures. Some value the caesarean as safer for their baby even if it may not be for them.

Informed choice

Some women choose to investigate birth in detail and their preference is based on a personal assessment of risk. For example, a large scale research programme in 2006 specifically comparing VBAC with planned repeat caesarean found "that a trial of labour by women with a history of caesarean delivery is associated with an increased risk of adverse perinatal outcomes and a higher rate of maternal adverse events, as compared with elective repeated caesarean delivery. The magnitude of these risks is small; however, this information is important for women and health care providers who are making choices about the type of delivery." (Professor Mark Landon, Chair of Obstetrics and Gynaecology, Ohio State University[246]) Women reviewing such research may develop specific opinions on issues such as: safety and risks associated with mode of delivery, availability of appropriate staff or likely outcomes for their situation. Sara Paterson-Brown Consultant Obstetrician, Queen Charlotte's and Chelsea Hospital, London says "Can we do all this [referring to increased safety of caesarean procedure, family planning, antenatal screening, prenatal counselling etc.] and then refuse a woman a safe mode of delivery (caesarean section) that removes the gambles associated with labour and which she personally finds unacceptable?"[247] For some women such research points them toward a request for a *prophylactic* caesarean in order to avoid labour or the risks of other forms of medical intervention including an unplanned caesarean.

Level of healthcare available

Standards of care, expertise and staff availability vary within countries and between hospitals. Awareness of this may encourage some women to approach specific hospitals and make specific birthing choices. This is particularly likely if they have been told or assume their birth may be more complex and require greater expertise.

Preserve pelvic floor and sexual experience

Some women believe that a caesarean will protect their pelvic floor and reduce the impact of birth on subsequent sexual experience. Pregnancy itself plays a significant part in pelvic floor issues and a caesarean does not entirely remove the likelihood of pelvic floor problems (see Appendix C). Such a request is unlikely to be accepted in isolation.

Social convenience

This term is often viewed negatively but actually encompasses many reasons, some of which will be more accepted than others. A single mother with other children and no family support network may benefit from planning the exact timing of her birth, enabling her to arrange childcare and home support for herself and her children. A mother simply wanting to fit in with a busy social calendar is likely to have more difficulty gaining agreement.

> *"As a woman wanting children in the future I am already terrified of the physical and emotional impact on my body in general. I'd like to have the option to have a birth that I want and not one that's dictated to me by doctors or midwives." Elizabeth (32)*

The benefits and risks of caesarean and vaginal birth

The following information considers the possible negative outcomes of caesareans (planned or otherwise) and medicalised vaginal births as well as the benefits of more straightforward experiences. As discussed throughout the book the preference for a straightforward, natural vaginal birth is just that, a preference and not something that can be guaranteed. In the same way, a planned caesarean is a preference too and complications can arise. In both cases try not to be alarmed at the long list of possible complications, the rarity of many of these is clearly indicated in each section.

Benefits in common

The following benefits are common to both vaginal births and planned caesareans under regional anaesthetic (unplanned caesareans under regional anaesthetic *may* also afford the following benefits):

Awake and alert

Unless you have experienced a protracted laboured or require a general anaesthetic during a caesarean you will be fully conscious and able to hold / feed your baby straight away. In the case of a planned caesarean you should be able to do both certainly in the recovery room if not in theatre.

Immediate skin-to-skin and eye contact

This is incredibly reassuring for your baby and possible with both types of birth. In the case of a caesarean you need to agree this in advance as it can be quite difficult to manage due to the constraints of the screen, gown etc.

Breastfeeding

Your baby can breastfeed immediately unless medical complications indicate otherwise. After a caesarean this again needs to be with prior agreement so the screen and your gown can be positioned accordingly.

Birth partner present

Your birth partner can be with you at all times unless significant difficulties arise requiring a general anaesthetic, in which case they may be asked to step outside for a time.

Benefits of a caesarean birth

For you

Safety

Where a complex birth is predicted a planned caesarean may be the safest option. Similarly, pregnancy or labour may suddenly alter making an unplanned caesarean now safer than continuing with a vaginal attempt.

Speed

Quicker than most vaginal deliveries, a caesarean takes less than an hour and this can be crucial in an emergency situation.

Controlled

Where medical reasons suggest delivery needs to be controlled, e.g. problems with the placenta, HIV transmission etc., a planned caesarean can offer a more manageable environment.[248][249]

Dedicated team

Every expert you or your baby could need is on hand throughout surgery and for at least an hour afterwards.

Prophylactic choice

A planned caesarean removes many of the unpredictable risks associated with vaginal birth, which can be particularly significant for more complex births (see Chapter 3 & Appendix B).

An emotional high

The sense of achievement and emotional high associated with the arrival of your baby can be significant particularly if labour, with its accompanying hormone rush, has initiated delivery.

Avoidance of labour

The ability to avoid labour can be very important for women needing to manage significant levels of fear (tokophobia) or those who have experienced abuse,[250] previous traumatic vaginal birth or female genital mutilation.[251]

Vaginal protection

The vagina is not damaged unless you have first laboured for a prolonged period or an instrumental delivery has been attempted.

Intercourse

The chances are sexual intercourse will resume sooner after a caesarean than following a vaginal birth,[252] with less pain associated.[253]

Timing

Surgery can be arranged to coincide with other factors e.g. availability of birth partner, support networks for siblings, work commitments etc.

Pelvic floor protection

This is often assumed to be a benefit of caesarean birth but while it reduces the likelihood of problems it cannot guarantee this. Stress incontinence has typically been associated with vaginal delivery, particularly episiotomy and instrumental deliveries.[254] However, the debate also suggests being pregnant (weight carried for a prolonged period) and increasing age may also cause a weakening of these muscles over time. Practitioners cannot agree, though there is evidence to suggest a reduction in such problems following caesarean deliveries.[255]

For your baby

Many of the benefits to you also apply to your baby.

Birth timing

The caesarean can be planned for a point in time deemed safer for your baby, avoiding risks which may be present if your baby is carried to term, e.g. in the case of specific medical conditions.

Safety

Complex situations can be managed as they arise.

Speed

See above.

Dedicated team

See above.

Benefits of a vaginal birth

For you

Drug free

By limiting drugs to no more than gas and air you can manage drug related side effects for you and your baby.

Continuity of care

You may have the same midwife with you throughout your birth, building up trust and confidence. This cannot be guaranteed by many hospitals, but is more likely with midwife-led units and independent midwives.

An emotional high

The rush of hormones following vaginal birth can create a high so significant it has been likened to *falling in love.*

A mum commenting on her vaginal birth said "I do not really remember the pain, and what I can remember felt very positive, each pain bringing me closer to my baby." Carol (29)

Home birth

You may be able to labour and deliver in the reassuring comfort of your own home or at least labour at home for quite some time before going into hospital.

Lower blood loss

In an average, straightforward birth this is lower than during a caesarean.

Faster physical recovery

For those experiencing a straightforward, instrument-free birth, recovery can be quick.

Sense of achievement and fulfilment

By following your natural human instincts you may feel a tremendous sense of achievement.

Going home

You can leave hospital the same day, if all goes well.

For your baby

Many of the benefits to you also apply to your baby, she will be: awake, alert, potentially drug-free, able to breastfeed. In addition:

Born when she is ready

Unless you are induced your baby will be born when she is ready to be. You will both experience the hormonal changes that are a natural, useful part of birth. For example, labour activates the mechanism to absorb lung fluid more quickly.

Lung health

Passage down the birth canal compresses your baby's chest expelling excess fluid from the lungs.

Comparison of the risks

The list of risks for both caesarean and vaginal birth looks lengthy but includes possibilities in their worse case scenarios, many of which are actually very rare.

IMPORTANT: A VBAC carries additional risks to those listed in Vaginal birth risks (see Chapter 6). Take these into consideration when planning a VBAC.

Caesarean birth risks (to Mum)

Delivery pain

While regional anaesthesia ensures you do not feel sharp pain you are likely to feel a *rummaging* (pulling and tugging) sensation. This can be rather vigorous and disconcerting but for most is not generally painful. A general anaesthetic puts you completely to sleep and you do not experience any delivery pain or sensation but nor are you aware of your baby's birth (see Risks with anaesthetics, in this chapter).

Blood loss

You may lose more blood during a caesarean than a straightforward vaginal birth but any resulting anaemia can be treated. Where blood loss cannot be controlled, a transfusion may be necessary. This is extremely rare, particularly for planned caesareans [256] [257] [258] (63 in 10,000 caesareans require transfusion according to one study[259]) and are generally associated with underlying medical conditions[260] e.g. placenta accrete, placenta praevia etc.[261]

Medical intervention

A caesarean is of course medical intervention in itself (see Caesarean birth – Delivery injuries, in this chapter). Very rarely forceps (through the incision – not the vaginal) may be required if your baby has become stuck (see Vaginal birth – Medical intervention, in this chapter).

Blood clots (Deep Vein Thrombosis – DVT)

This is very rare, though a possibility in any pregnancy (1 in 1,000) but surgery increases the incidence. It occurs in approximately 4-16 in every 10,000 caesareans.[262] Surgical stockings and blood thinning injections reduce this risk.

Scar rupture

The risk of a caesarean scar rupturing during pregnancy is very low and the risk of this happening during a repeat caesarean is extremely low (12 in 10,000).[263]

Delivery injury

The incision cuts through skin and muscle and some damage will result, more so with a classical incision (vertical cut). The incision will be red, a little swollen and sore for a week or so but the incision itself *should* seal within 12 hours. You will find moving about quite challenging in the first 24 hours as muscles are damaged. Over the next week the pain is managed with medication and as long as you move with care, avoiding sudden movements and unnecessary strain, it can be managed or avoided. Muscles will repair and with light exercise (after the 6 week check) full muscle tone *should* return.

A caesarean scar fades with time but is unlikely to disappear entirely. For some it becomes a flat, fine, pale line, for others a ridge will remain and it may continue to be sensitive (not painful) to touch for some time. Some women do find that *puffiness* remains immediately above the scar and for those carrying more weight this can appear like a skin fold, however for many women this disappears with time.

Most caesarean scars are horizontal. Vertical incisions are rare (less than 1 in 100)[266] and only used in specific circumstances e.g. a very large or premature baby or a baby lying across the uterus (transverse). However in this instance the scar will be visible above your bikini line.

In addition to the incision scar, nearby organs (e.g. bladder and bowel) may be damaged. Such incidents are rare, for example 1 in 1,000 suffer a bladder injury,[267] even less frequent with

> **Natural childbirth**
>
> This is "a philosophy that is not universal, but rather the product of a particular subculture. [A study in 1986] concludes that C-section itself is not particularly emotionally traumatic, but has the power to be traumatic among women schooled in the rhetoric of *natural* childbirth." Dr Margarete Sandelowski, Women's health specialist at University of North Carolina[264]
> A recent commentator adds "it is the expectations encouraged by NCB [Natural Childbirth] philosophy that lead to these negative outcomes..." Dr. Amy Tuteur, Obstetrician &Gynaecologist[265]

planned, pre-labour caesareans and repair work is carried out during the caesarean.

Negative emotional reaction

Both vaginal and caesarean births[268] [269] have the potential to cause emotional distress, particularly when a birth does not go to plan or the experience does not match a mother's expectations. This can be severe for some women and require treatment (see Appendix D).

Death

Extremely rare. Figures vary but the trend suggests the risk of death is fractionally lower for planned, pre-labour caesareans (31 deaths per 1,000,000) [270] [271] than for vaginal birth (which includes those ending with unplanned caesareans where medical complications necessitate intervention).[272] [273]

Staff and facility shortages

Planned caesareans can be affected by staff and facility availability. Caesareans require specific specialists and cannot begin until these are available. The number of theatres is limited in most hospitals and emergencies take precedence. Similarly, anaesthetists are a stretched resource as they are supporting labouring women too and this may also delay planned caesareans.

Invasion of privacy

Surgery requires a specific number of people (12 typically) and you may feel intimidated or disappointed with the public nature of your birth.

Vaginal birth risks (to Mum)

Delivery pain

Experiences vary but for most, labour and delivery is very painful. While some perceive it as positive pain, for others fear, exhaustion and tension can alter hormone levels, physically increasing pain to a point where pain relief is requested. Epidurals will remove the pain but *should not* remove the sensation of labour and delivery. UK figures in 2008-09 show a third of NHS hospital vaginal births include anaesthetic during labour.[274]

Blood loss

This will occur in a straightforward vaginal delivery and can lead to temporary anaemia, which can be treated if severe, though the need for a transfusion is rare. Medical intervention (i.e. forceps), increases the likelihood of greater bleeding[275] and sometimes blood loss may need to be controlled with drugs.

Medical intervention

Some form of intervention is used in over 50% of UK hospital based vaginal births.[276]

- **Ventouse and/or forceps** – Rates are significant, reportedly between 12 in 100[277] and 23 in 100.[278] While sometimes crucial in a difficult vaginal birth, these instruments are invasive and can physically damage both you and your baby (see – this chapter). The need for repair work to your vaginal area is likely. [More info.[xx]] In addition to increased risk of infection and excessive blood loss, instrumental deliveries are associated with increased risk of bowel problems, urinary and anal incontinence, haemorrhoids, pain during sex and severe emotional reactions. Women report the latter can affect their ability to bond with and breastfeed their baby. The amount of damage can be perceived as greater than a caesarean and certainly more than a straightforward vaginal birth,[279] affecting movement and causing significant pain during recovery. Ventouse seem to cause less damage and pain to you than forceps,[280] with forceps particularly linked to increased incidence of pelvic floor issues. There is some suggestion that women should be counselled to consider a caesarean rather than forceps intervention when experiencing a birth that requires instrumental assistance[281]

- **Episiotomy** – This surgical cut to the perineum (the area between your vagina and anus) requires stitching after delivery and can make sitting and walking difficult for several weeks. The impact on your sex life may last longer. 13 in 100 UK women have an episiotomy.[282] Having an episiotomy will not reduce the chances of third and fourth degree tears.[283] An episiotomy *should not* be conducted routinely for instrumental deliveries but reserved for situations of acute fetal distress

- **Epidurals** – Their rate of use in labour varies between hospitals. Some hospitals record rates well above 50%.[284] [285] Epidurals take 20 minutes to set up and a further 20 minutes to take effect so are not generally used in the late stages of labour – timing your request so you do not leave it too late can be difficult, they can feel essential for some women (see Risks with anaesthetics, in this chapter)

- **Induction** – If your pregnancy extends beyond 41 weeks you risk being induced. Induction is an intervention used to start labour e.g. manually breaking waters, administering artificial chemicals etc.:

  - A clear link has been established between induction and an increase in medical intervention (instruments, anaesthetics and caesarean). 20% of births are induced[286]

[xx] www.ukpmc.ac.uk search for Farrell Cesarean section versus forceps-assisted vaginal birth

- Contractions may be more severe and if chemicals are used and dosages too high there will be no wax and wane of pain, rather your contractions begin at their peak rendering gas and air less effective [More info.[xxi]] increasing the likelihood of you requesting an epidural

- The contractions can cause fetal distress due to their frequency and strength, again leading to further medical intervention

- There is an increased risk of uterine rupture where there have been previous caesareans[287 288 289]

- A miscalculation of due dates can result in a premature birth and lower APGAR scores. Calculating the size of your baby is not an exact science and due dates should not be used in isolation when making a decision to induce

- If the two of you are really not ready you may still not go into labour but you and baby will have been flooded with artificial hormones

- **Unplanned caesarean** – Approximately 25% of all UK births (33% in the US) end with a caesarean delivery. Over half of these are classed *emergency*. The physical and particularly the emotional impact of unplanned caesareans can be significant (see Chapter 1 & Appendix D)

DVT

There is a risk of developing a blood clot with any pregnancy (1 in 1,000). Surgical stockings which can help prevent this are not generally provided unless you are at particularly high risk.

Scar rupture

The likelihood of a previous caesarean scar rupturing is higher during a VBAC (35 in 10,000)[290] than a repeat caesarean and some practitioners automatically recommend a repeat caesarean on this basis. Figures vary [291] [292] but the trend is consistent though overall the incidence is low. The risk of fetal death as a result of a scar rupture is very low (45 in 100,000) but again higher than for a planned caesarean.[293]

Scar separations can be minor (scar *dehiscence*) but when planning a VBAC it is important you know the type of incision made at your previous caesarean. Rupture rates increase fractionally with vertical *uterus* incisions (2-4 in 100).[294] Remember, the external scar is not necessarily the orientation of your internal scar. Rupture rates also increase with the number of caesareans you have[295] and induction has been shown to increase the risks to "80 per 10,000 if non-prostaglandins are used, 240 per

---

[xxi] www.nice.org.uk search for Induction of labour

10,000 if prostaglandins are used" after previous caesareans. (UK NICE caesarean guideline[296])

Delivery injury

Where tears or cuts to the vagina, perineum and/or anus occur repair will be required in all except first degree tears and some second degree tears. 85-90% of women will tear.[297] In the US, 52% of mothers report having been stitched.[298] Repair work is usually carried out in the delivery room but third and fourth degree tears will require anaesthetic and you may be moved to theatre and potentially separated from your baby. Such injury will slow your recovery (see Vaginal birth – Medical intervention, in this chapter).

Death

Extremely rare (39 deaths per 1,000,000 vaginal births and unplanned caesarean births).[299] [300] Maternal deaths overall are generally associated with the underlying medical condition (thrombosis and pre-eclampsia being the primary causes) and not the caesarean itself.[301]

Staff shortages

Midwifery services can be overstretched on any given day and you may labour alone for significant periods.[302] The recommended ratio of midwives to labouring women is 1 to 1.15[303] but with staff shortages common, even in the developed world, this is difficult to achieve outside of homebirths or midwife-led units. Unfortunately, midwifery shortages (10,000 in the UK) can mean that your midwife may actually be caring for 3-5 women at the same time.[304] [More info.[xxii]] Similarly, anaesthetists are a stretched resource, particularly at night, and your pain relief may be late or absent entirely.

Variable facilities

Unless you are giving birth in a midwife-led unit with facilities and staff guaranteed, a birth pool may be unavailable when you want it and at busy times individual rooms for delivery may be full. The size of your hospital will determine the number of postnatal beds and at busy times it may be that you are encouraged to go home after your birth before you feel ready.

Invasion of privacy

Unless you give birth at home or in a midwife-led unit you may be attended by 10 or more individuals during your labour. Not all at the same time[305] and many will be unknown to you.

---

xxii www.rcm.org.uk search for Baby boom and midwife shortages

Caesarean birth risks (to baby)

Injuries

Cuts are very rare, occurring in 7 in 1,000 caesareans. [306] They are typically connected with emergencies where the speed of delivery, type of incision and the reason for the surgery play a part.[307] The likelihood increases if the uterus is contracting[308] but the majority are skin lacerations from a sterile scalpel and have no long term consequences.

Breathing difficulties

Babies born prematurely may encounter breathing difficulties requiring admission to SCU. Planning a caesarean for week 39 reduces the level of risk to no longer statistically significantly different to that of vaginal birth at the same stage.[309] For this reason official guidelines recommend caesareans not be scheduled before 39 weeks, when the lungs are fully mature, unless medically necessary.[310] [311] Many studies acknowledge that both prematurity[312] [313] [314] [315] and the underlying reason for the caesarean play a significant part in the likelihood of experiencing breathing difficulties. It *may be* that caesareans without labour increase risk[316] but research is unclear on this specific point. What is clear is that the later your caesarean, the lower the risk.

Delayed breastfeeding

There is no reason to delay feeding except: where your health is so compromised that breastfeeding is impossible or in cases of general anaesthetic where you may both be still asleep or too drowsy to feed. However it is often assumed you will feed once in the recovery room or later still once back on the postnatal ward. In actual fact with a regional anaesthetic you *may* be able to breastfeed while still in theatre. While there is no long-term impact upon the likelihood of your still feeding at 8 months[317] any short delay can feel disappointing and birth trauma can increase stress hormones affecting lactation (see Chapter 6).

Prematurity

Aside from instances where medical conditions indicate early delivery, the main reason for prematurity is incorrect due dates. Check them thoroughly before confirming your caesarean and avoid scheduling it before 39 weeks unless medically necessary (see Caesarean birth risks – Breathing difficulties, in this chapter).

Anaesthetics

See Risks with anaesthetic.

Asthma

Research connecting baby's development of asthma to caesareans is contradictory and inconclusive. Studies find either no link[318] [319] or included *significant* additional factors such as prematurity, maternal asthma,[320] allergic parents,[321] being born with respiratory difficulties etc.[322]

Development of beneficial gut bacteria

Your baby's gut becomes colonised with *good* bacteria in her first week. For babies born by caesarean this process may take longer and result in an increase in diarrhoea for a short time. However, more than a quarter of caesarean births are before 40 weeks and the reasons for the early birth may actually delay colonisation rather than the caesarean itself.

Admission to SCU

Most admissions to SCU are related to the underlying reason for the caesarean. Planned caesareans prior to 39 weeks seem to account for *some* of these.[323]

Death

This is very rare and rarely the fault of the caesarean but rather the underlying medical condition requiring such intervention.[324] In the case of repeat caesareans the rate is 1 in 10,000.[325]

Vaginal birth risks (to baby)

Injuries

12 in 100 UK births involve forceps or ventouse. The overall risk of injury is *very* small for each of the following:

- **Instrument injury** - Facial injuries and severe bruising following instrumental delivery[326]

- **Nerve damage** to the face, eyes, arms and shoulder. The effect is usually temporary. In longer term and more severe cases, surgery can improve outcomes. Incidence is 24 in 1,000 (forceps), 32 in 1,000 (ventouse). [327] Of these 1 in 100 may suffer permanent damage[328]

- **Bleeding** inside the baby's skull (haemorrhage)[329]

[More info.[xxiii]]

[xxiii] www.nejm.org search for Towner nejm Effect of mode of delivery

Breathing difficulties

In the case of a premature or difficult birth your baby may have respiratory difficulties and need to wear an oxygen mask to receive extra oxygen. In some cases she may require admission to SCU.

Delayed breastfeeding

There is no reason to delay feeding except: in cases of extreme exhaustion, your health being so compromised that breastfeeding is impossible or your baby being asleep.

Prematurity

Some babies do come early and your baby may need to spend time in SCU.

Anaesthetic

Opiates (e.g. pethidine and diamorphine) cross the placenta and are present in breast milk, this can make your baby drowsy and uninterested in feeding for a time. Regional anaesthetics do not affect your baby's alertness (see Risks with anaesthetics, in this chapter).

Admission to SCU

Where complications arise prior to or during vaginal birth, some babies will need additional support for a time and this may require admission to SCU.

Death

Very rare, approximately 10 in 10,000, the same risk as for a VBAC.[330]

Anaesthetics

A third of UK vaginal births use anaesthesia at some point.[331] Even if you hope to avoid a caesarean or plan to birth without an epidural it is worth understanding anaesthetics in advance as you may find yourself asking for one on the day. There will be little time for detailed questions at such a late stage.

Benefits of anaesthetics

There is a description of anaesthetics is in Chapter 1. [More info.[xxiv]]

Regional anaesthetic (epidural and spinal only)

- **Numb** – The chest, abdomen and legs are numbed. Your arms are not and you can hold your baby immediately

---

[xxiv] www.oaa.anaes.ac.uk search for Your anaesthetic for caesarean section

- **Awake** – You can see and hear everything. You will not be sleepy and may be able to feed your baby in theatre
- **Effect on baby** – Little to no effect[332] [333]
- **Safe** – Very safe
- **Birth partner** – Present

General anaesthetic

- **Speed** – You will be asleep within 5 minutes and distress and pain will subside almost immediately. Your baby is delivered very quickly, crucial in critical situations

Risks with anaesthetics

Unless otherwise stated the following risks refer to mum.

Regional anaesthetic

- **Sickness** – Caused by a drop in blood pressure during surgery – this is quite common (1 in 5).[334] Tell your anaesthetist as drugs administered through your IV can quickly remove the sensation
- **Severe headache** – Occurs in less than 1 in 100 epidurals and in even fewer with a spinal.[335] While very severe it is treatable
- **Itchiness** – Generally around the face and quite common – treatable if severe
- **Extended numbness** – The *block* may rise higher than intended making you feel breathless, though your breathing is not actually impaired
- **Nerve damage** – Temporary numb patches remaining on your skin are quite common. Occasionally women experience temporary leg weakness (1 in 1,000). It is very rare for this to be permanent (1 in 13,000),[336] perhaps even lower (1 in 300,000).[337] Severe injury resulting in paralysis is extremely rare (1 in 250,000)[338]
- **Sensation returns early** – Sensation may return earlier than expected. This is very rare and an epidural can be topped up if needed
- **Effect on your baby** – Small amounts of anaesthetic cross the placenta, however, it does not have an adverse affects on your baby[339]

General anaesthetic

General anaesthetic has a number of additional risks associated. For this reason it is only used where a regional is not possible. In addition to the risks already outlined for regional anaesthetics, you should take account of the following:

- **Respiratory complications for mum** – This is rare and caused by stomach acids flowing back from the stomach into the lungs leading to pneumonia (1 in 300)[340]

- **Awareness** – The risk of awareness during surgery is extremely rare. If it does occur it is typically awareness of voices and movement rather than pain[341] (1 in 14,000)[342]

- **Chest infection** – While common (1 in 5), most infections are not severe[343] and can be treated with antibiotics that do not affect breast milk

- **Anaphylaxis** – Severe allergic reaction to the anaesthetic is extremely rare (1 in 10-20,000)[344]

- **Death** – Extremely rare, less than 1 in 100,000, i.e. 1-2 a year in the UK[345]

- **Drowsiness and sickness** – You are likely to feel drowsy but there is a possibility that you may also feel sick as you wake (1 in 10).[346] It can take several hours for the nausea to wear off so ask your midwife for something to counteract this

- **Effect on your baby** – The drugs used will cross the placenta and are likely to make her drowsy in the short term. This may initially affect her ability and interest in feeding

- **Skin-to-skin and breastfeeding** – Being asleep, you will be unable to breastfeed or actively hold your baby skin-to-skin for several hours (though your partner can place your baby next to your skin and support her there or hold her skin-to-skin himself)

- **Emotional negativity** – You are not awake when she is born and it can be several hours before you meet her. This can be distressing and some women connect this delay to bonding difficulties

- **Alone** – Your birth partner will not be with you when you are put to sleep and is unlikely to be present during surgery. They will be left alone with no news of you or your baby for some time

Recovery

Caesarean birth recovery

Pain and mobility

Incision pain should be expected for up to a week, longer if there is infection. Medication makes the pain manageable in most cases but does not remove it entirely, particularly if you make sudden movements or over extend yourself. You will feel rather slow on your feet and will find getting out of bed and chairs uncomfortable for 2-3 days. Following this you will need to move with care for several weeks to avoid sharp pain associated with twisting or straining the incision area. If pain persists after 4 weeks seek guidance.

Infection

Largely preventable through pre-operative medication and scrupulous postoperative care but the incidence is approximately 6 in 100.[347] Infection is treated with antibiotics compatible with breastfeeding but these can interfere with baby's digestive system temporarily.

Pelvic floor problems

A planned caesarean cannot absolutely remove the chance of pelvic floor problems but can reduce them by avoiding the need for instrumental delivery. [More info.[xxv]]

Tiredness

If you have laboured first you are more likely to be tired. However the emotional rollercoaster of a baby's arrival can make you feel very tired in any case, particularly after the initial euphoria wears off.

Drug-related drowsiness

See Risks with anaesthetics.

Duration

While surgery itself is typically no more than an hour this can increase (by minutes not hours) if you have scar tissue from previous surgery or if repair work is required (e.g. to bowel or bladder).

[xxv] www.prlog.org search for McDonagh Hull Pelvic floor protection

Difficulty breastfeeding

Breastfeeding can be hard to establish with any birth experience, but getting into position following a caesarean can be an added problem and baby kicks on the incision are uncomfortable. Stress hormones may affect your ability to breastfeed (see Vaginal birth – Negative emotional response, in this chapter and Chapter 6). However specialists *should* be available to help you.

Negative emotional response

Unplanned caesareans or planned caesareans that encounter difficulties can leave you traumatised. At its mildest this may be feelings of disappointment, but for some major depression or post-traumatic stress disorder (PTSD) can result, affecting bonding and your ability to cope with the challenges of motherhood. In such cases counselling may be needed. If severe it can cause a woman to avoid becoming pregnant again.

Constipation

Your digestive tract slows following surgery. Constipation is a common side effect of anaesthetic (coupled with increased immobility). This can cause mild to severe discomfort and can be distressing when trying to go to the toilet. It can be eased through appropriate diet and medication if severe.

Trapped gas

A side effect of surgery, it can be painful if not dislodged, though drinking peppermint tea can help.

Scarring and swelling

The closure technique, your skin type and your weight pre and post birth play a part in the appearance of the scar area. With time it should become a pale white line though for some it continues as a slightly raised red line. For some women *puffiness* may remain above the scar due to a combination of weight, muscle tone, skin type etc. but for most this will again disappear with time.

Women of mainly African origin may develop keloid scarring. These occur when the naturally occurring scar tissue continues to grow creating a raised scar that is hard to the touch. While not generally painful they can remain red or purple for some time. Susceptibility to keloid scarring tends to run in families.

Reduced muscle tone

Surgery cuts some stomach muscle. The extent is kept to a minimum, many surgeons preferring to use a small cut from which they tear long muscle groups. Most uterus incisions are horizontal but in rare cases where a vertical incision is needed muscles are more effected. Careful exercise can generally fully restore muscle tone.

Hospital stay

A hospital stay will be necessary, typically 2-4 days, and is dependent upon baby's health and feeding success as well as your recovery.

Intercourse

Discomfort following birth may cause you to feel less interested in sex and may continue as a significant barrier for weeks or months afterwards. Pain during intercourse is less likely than following a vaginal birth.

Recovery timescales

Your recovery will take longer than a straightforward vaginal birth with no tearing. Full recovery from a caesarean with no infection can be as little as 3-4 weeks but physical strain and poor post-operative cleanliness can extend this.

Endometritis (inflammation of the uterus wall)

While treatable, it can develop after a caesarean and lead to fever, abdominal pain and abnormal vaginal discharge. Rates vary between studies[348] and prophylactic antibiotics (now frequently used in caesareans) can significantly reduce the risk of this condition.

Repeat caesarean

Concerns about scar rupture amongst other things, means that a caesarean may be automatically offered for your subsequent births. This need not be the case and increasingly women are encouraged to labour (VBAC).

Vaginal birth recovery

Pain and mobility

Perineal pain is very likely after a vaginal birth, particularly following an instrumental delivery. Experiences vary but walking, sitting, intercourse and going to the toilet are likely to be painful in the first couple of weeks or for some women even months, particularly where instruments, episiotomies and tears have occurred or infection has set in.

Infection

Wound related infection is a possibility and there is an increased risk of infection where medical interventions (forceps, episiotomies etc.) are involved.[349] Affected areas may require further treatment.

Pelvic floor problems

These show, when coughing, sneezing or laughing and include urinary and bowel incontinence as well as leaking gas. It can also lead to changes in sexual sensation. While vaginal birth seems to increase the likelihood of pelvic floor problems, particularly where forceps are involved, it is not the only factor. Obesity, smoking, HRT and hysterectomies are also thought to be factors, as is the extra weight of pregnancy itself exerting pressure on these muscles. [More info.[xxvi]]

Tiredness

Some vaginal births can be very protracted causing severe exhaustion, particularly those involving instrumental delivery. With the best will in the world you may have little or no interest in your baby until you have slept.

Drug-related drowsiness

Some forms of pain relief (opiates such as pethidine or diamorphine) can affect you and your baby and your success with breastfeeding. For regional anaesthetic effects see Risks with anaesthetics.

Duration

Labour duration varies significantly from one woman to another and from one birth to the next, though subsequent labours tend to be quicker. It may be anything from several days to as little as several hours (particularly for subsequent labours).

Difficulty breastfeeding

Changes to stress hormones as a result of *any* type of traumatic birth (including protracted labour, instrumental birth or unplanned caesarean) can delay lactation.[350] [351] Breastfeeding can be hard to establish with even the most straightforward birth but those experiencing physical or emotional trauma may find it more difficult to keep on trying.[352] Specialists *should* be available to help you.

Negative emotional response

Emotional trauma can be associated with *any* complicated birth, particularly those involving interventions e.g. instrumental vaginal births.[353] It can have such a negative effect that it leads to avoidance of subsequent pregnancies[354] and may affect your desire to breastfeed[355] as well as your overall mood and ability to cope with motherhood.

Even straightforward vaginal births can feel negative,[356] but particularly so when preconceptions about birth do not match the experience.[357]

[xxvi] www.prlog.org search for McDonagh Hull Pelvic floor protection

Constipation

Medication can be used to counteract severe cases. Constipation can be very distressing the first few times you go to the toilet, particularly if you have open wounds or stitches.

Haemorrhoids

A potentially painful outcome of pregnancy and more often associated with vaginal birth. Creams and suppositories can reduce the swelling but they can be very difficult to get rid of, making sitting and going to the toilet a painful experience for quite some time.

Scarring and swelling

Where an episiotomy or tear has occurred swelling may be increased and will take several weeks to heal, or longer in more severe cases or where infection has set in. If treated promptly, this can be reduced. Indeed, swelling will occur after vaginal delivery in most cases, but more so after an instrumental delivery. If there has been prolonged pushing, labial and perineal swelling is more likely and haemorrhoids may be exacerbated making sitting and going to the toilet difficult. Ice and anti-inflammatories may be necessary.

An extended tear with a difficult vaginal delivery can involve the anal sphincter and immediate surgery is required. A follow up appointment at 10 to 12 weeks is necessary to assess whether any permanent damage has been done to the anal sphincter tone.

Reduced muscle tone

The prolonged stretching of abdominal muscles from the weight carried during pregnancy affects muscle tone for a time. Appropriate exercise can fully restore muscle tone.

Hospital stay

If your birth has been straightforward you can leave hospital within 12 hours, though injuries can double this time. Some women feel that this is too soon if they need extra support or are returning to a busy home environment.

Intercourse

Discomfort following birth may cause you to feel less interested in sex and it may continue as a significant barrier for weeks or months afterwards. However sexual relations may take longer to resume[358] and pain during intercourse is more likely after a vaginal birth than after a caesarean.[359]

Recovery timescales

Protracted births or those involving medical intervention will take longer to recover from (often as a long as a caesarean – 3-4 weeks). Unnecessary physical strain and poor post-delivery cleanliness can extend this.

Endometritis (inflammation of the uterus wall)

While treatable, it can develop after a vaginal birth and lead to fever, abdominal pain and abnormal vaginal discharge. Rates vary between studies.[360]

The implications of caesareans on future births

There are a number of implications of caesareans on future pregnancies. You should take these into account when considering any caesarean, particularly if you are planning a large family.

For you

Medical conditions causing complications

The occurrence of placenta praevia and placenta accreta increases with each caesarean[361] and can cause significant complications in subsequent births (see – this chapter). Women having a first caesarean are "2.6 times more likely to develop placenta praevia" (Maureen Connolly, Birth Commentator[362] et al) in a subsequent pregnancy. The incidence of placenta accreta is approximately 1 in 2,500 pregnancies[363] and appears to be associated with approximately 10% of placenta praevia cases.[364] Placenta accreta accounts for around 50% of unplanned hysterectomies.[365] While these conditions can occur without previous surgery (for example – placenta accreta occurs in 45 in 1,000 pregnancies without prior uterine surgery),[366] the more caesareans you have the greater the likelihood.[367]

Scar rupture

The risk of a caesarean scar rupturing during future pregnancies is very low. For horizontal scars the risk is so low that alone this should not be used as a reason against a VBAC (see Vaginal birth risks – Scar rupture, in this chapter).

Longer surgery

Scar tissue and adhesions from previous surgery can extend surgery time and complexity.

Infertility and avoidance of subsequent pregnancies

This is an on-going debate and more research is needed before definite conclusions with regards the impact of caesarean and instrumental vaginal delivery (IVD) can be made. Some evidence suggests that pelvic infections and internal scars following both *may* impact fertility[368] [369] and increase the incidence of ectopic pregnancies,[370] while others suggest that IVD is not implicated[371] and that *uncomplicated* caesareans do not appear to lead to tubal infertility.[372] [373] [374] Studies also show that, on average, a longer gap occurs between pregnancies after a caesarean birth compared to women with no previous caesarean delivery[375] and that emotional trauma may contribute to this.[376] [377] Most studies have also gone on to include caveats concerning *voluntary* infertility following caesareans and IVD. They suggest that birth trauma can, consciously or sub-consciously, delay couples getting pregnant again or indeed cause them to avoid further pregnancies. [378] [379] [380] [381] [382] This question over the extent to which social and psychological factors may impact fertility highlights the importance of learning about and preparing for the possibility of caesareans and developing realistic attitudes to this form of intervention in particular.

Ectopic pregnancies

Here the egg implants outside the uterus. This is very rare and not conclusively connected with caesareans. Where it does occur a termination is necessary and there is a risk of severe bleeding requiring surgery.[383]

Number of caesareans

There is no limit to the number of caesareans you can have though the increasing risk of medical complications and scar tissue formation etc. suggests that where possible vaginal birth would be preferable if you are planning a large family.

Frequency of pregnancies

There is no clear guideline for this in relation to the risk of scar rupture. While greatest in birth with small gaps between, scar rupture is still relatively rare.[384] [385] [386] Social and psychological factors may have implications on the frequency of planned pregnancies (see Future births – Infertility, in this chapter).

For your baby

Death

Extremely rare (10 in 10,000 VBACs),[387] lower still (1 in 10,000) with a planned repeat caesarean.[388] Other reports show the same trend.[389]

Stillbirth

Research has looked at whether there is a link between previous caesareans and stillbirth in a subsequent pregnancy. Results are contradictory and "it is not possible to disentangle the effect of CS from the reasons for CS." (UK NICE caesarean guideline[390]) The following studies were reviewed during the research for this sub-topic.[391] [392] [393] [394] [395]

Clinical definitions of difficult reactions

If you think that you are experiencing any of the following you may benefit from additional support. Talk to your health visitors or doctor as they will be able to give you advice on where to get help, whether this is help around the home or with counselling.

Baby blues

Weepiness, tiredness and feeling tense can take you by surprise within a few days of your birth. This is common and can feel upsetting as it does not seem to fit with the joy of a new baby. Few women escape it entirely but for those that don't it generally does not last for more than a few weeks. At the time it is worrying as it can make you feel you are not coping or that you do not like your baby. *Baby blues* is thought to be triggered not just by hormonal changes but by the many physical, practical and financial changes that accompany your baby's arrival, and sleep deprivation does not help. People trying to jolly you out of it or telling you to pull yourself together are not helpful. Rest as much as you can, get as much support as you can and be assured it is common and will pass.

Postnatal depression (PnD)

Approximately 10%[396] of women suffer significant levels of postnatal depression. PnD is not confined to any particular culture or socioeconomic group[397] and can start at any time within the first year. The severity varies and it can be difficult to spot, particularly if you experienced significant baby blues. If you are exhibiting signs practitioners should be assessing you periodically looking at your levels of exhaustion, tearfulness, anxiety, sense of hopelessness and loneliness. Many women experience these feelings but with PnD they do not go away and your interest in caring for yourself will be likely to deteriorate. It is not certain what causes PnD. Some practitioners believe it is primarily hormonal imbalances associated with birth. Others believe physical and emotional challenges also play a part, such as lack of support and feelings of isolation, difficulties breastfeeding or ongoing health problems for you or your baby. [More info.xxvii] For women at risk of PnD a planned caesarean does not prevent it developing, but nor are unplanned caesareans more likely to cause PnD.[398] Keep in close touch with practitioners until you start to come out the other side. PnD is treatable and can be tackled in two distinct ways:

- Counselling often centres around a structured technique called Cognitive Behavioural Therapy (CBT) that helps develop strategies for coping with your specific symptoms, in particular negative thinking. By looking at your perceptions and thought processes and learning relaxation techniques you can re-think your birth. You may need a referral for such therapy and waiting lists can be long but there are a number of organisations specialising in helping women suffering from PnD (see Other resources). Finding others to support you can make a difference on a daily basis, in particular meeting other mothers. Organisations like the NCT and Meet a Mum are particularly good at facilitating this (see Other resources)

- Medication involves anti-depressants that can be used when breastfeeding. While these can be addictive and do have side effects the benefits can be noticeable within 2 weeks

Puerperal psychosis

This is a severe form of PnD. It is very rare (1 in 1,000 mothers)[399] and is characterised by manic, depressive and occasionally schizophrenic episodes sometimes accompanied by hallucinations or delusions. Its cause is thought to be sudden drops in pregnancy hormone levels (progesterone and oestrogen). Treatment is *essential* and needs hospitalisation, drug and ECT therapy for a period of 2-3 months.

Post Traumatic Stress Disorder (PTSD)

This is a rare, severe negative reaction to childbirth. The actual incidence is unknown but thought to affect 2 in 100 mothers.[400] It is caused by events during and surrounding birth e.g. medical emergencies and interventions, feelings of loss, absence of control and lack of partner support[401] [402] rather than hormonal changes. Unlike PnD it may be more likely in women with a history of tokophobia,[403] additional psychological difficulties or anxiety. The symptoms of PTSD are: vivid and highly distressing flashbacks, nightmares affecting sleep quality, feeling numb or detached from baby and partners/surroundings, avoidance of anything that might trigger birth memories including attending hospital or scenes on TV or prolonged, significant difficulties with sex and avoidance of further pregnancies. A mother talking about her birth and suffering from PTSD may use terms like

---

xxvii www.birthtraumaassociation.org.uk look up PTSD in 'Leaflets'

violation, abuse and even *rape*. Drugs are generally ineffective (though may be used as an anti-depressant to support recovery). Counselling is the usual treatment and CBT has been shown to be quite effective. [More info.[xxviii] [xxix]] Severe cases of PnD can be confused with PTSD and vice versa so that diagnoses are for a time inaccurate and treatment inappropriate. Here the regular support of practitioners is important and they should assess you over time. If you feel you are not getting the support you need keep asking and if necessary seek help from relevant voluntary organisations (see Other resources).

Paternal postnatal depression (PPnD)

As many as 1 in 14 men may suffer from depression before or after the birth of their baby.[404] Studies do not talk of female partner's susceptibility to PnD but it is reasonable to assume that, given female partners will experience the same pressures and worries before and after the birth that a male partner would, they are equally at risk. So, while I refer to this condition as PPnD to distinguish it here from PnD, consider that it is just as possible female partners may suffer from this condition too.

Symptoms to look for are:

- Feeling isolated

- Anger and increased irritability

- Lack of energy

- Sleeplessness (more than that associated with a newborn in the house)

- Anxiety attacks not necessarily related to baby

- Loss of sex drive

- Easily distracted

- Substance abuse as a coping technique

- Physical sensations such as headaches and stomach pains

In isolation each of these symptoms may be manageable however together and with increased levels they may indicate PPnD.

The triggers for PPnD vary from person to person, but in addition to those discussed in Chapter 7 (changes in lifestyle, isolation, increased responsibility, financial pressures, mis-matched birth expectations, trauma and Mum's depression[405]) your susceptibility is increased if you have had

---

[xxviii] www.babcp.org.uk

[xxix] www.birthtraumaassociation.org.uk

previous depressive episodes.[406] Men also experience significant hormonal changes in preparation for the birth of their child[407] (a drop in testosterone and an increase in oxytocin and oestrogen). Given that hormones affect Mum's mood and tendency towards depressive episodes, it is reasonable to assume the same is true for men though medical studies have yet to confirm the connection conclusively.

What studies do clearly show is that there is a connection between paternal depression and the incidence of behavioural and language difficulties in children.[408] Official bodies have called for improvements in antenatal education for partners and increased postnatal support, including further training for practitioners visiting the home. However, at present there is little formal support for birth partners so it is crucial you recognise the signs yourself and approach your doctor for advice.

Birth plan template

This template is concerned only with caesarean birth. While there is some overlap with vaginal birth plans, you should read more broadly to build a vaginal birth plan (see Other resources). The following is a guide – there may be points you do not find relevant or want to re-order based on strong preferences. For details regarding these points see Chapter 5 & Appendix A.

Remember these are all *preferences* to be *negotiated* with your practitioners.

If there are specific things you want to avoid, write "I do not consent to..." but be aware that in certain medical situations you may be advised to change your mind in the interest of your health or that of your baby.

Medical preferences

- A delivery date at 39 weeks plus (unless medical reasons indicate otherwise)
- Whether to labour, or not, before a planned caesarean
- Type of anaesthetic (regional or general)
- *Natural caesarean* (see Chapter 1)
- Catheter timing (insertion and removal)
- Cord cutting (who and when)
- Closure preference (stitch or staple)
- Vitamin K injection
- With a vaginal birth you may want to express when and why you would prefer to move to a caesarean (i.e. in what circumstances and what interventions should be tried before switching)

Experience preferences

- Birth partner(s) named
- Partner present during set-up

- Special needs (language, diet or religion)
- Surgery commentary or not
- Students present or not
- Arms, gown and screen positioned to facilitate holding and/or breastfeeding in theatre
- Baby's arrival (lights dimmed, silence)
- Skin-to-skin (how, who and when – cleaned first or not)
- Who discovers the sex of baby
- General anaesthetic (whether you want your birth partner to be waiting in the recovery room so they are present when you wake)
- Baby checks (when, where and what you would prefer to be done later by you)
- Who accompanies baby if she goes elsewhere
- Placenta (viewing and keeping)
- Baby's first clothes
- Baby care if you are under a general (holding, feeding etc.)
- Photographs/video
- Music
- Private room
- Debrief (before leaving hospital)

Feeding preferences

- Breast or bottle feeding
- First breastfeeding attempt (theatre/recovery room or ward)
- Use of artificial nipples and milk supplements (including water, sugar water or formula)
- Feeding preference if you have a general anaesthetic or your baby is in SCU (stored expressed milk)

Questions to ask your practitioners

The following list focuses on caesarean birth and is by no means exhaustive – view it as a starting point only.

HINTS:

- Be specific – e.g. *How often do you perform caesareans?* This is quite open ended and may not reveal the caesarean rate for the practitioner or the hospital, nor will it give you a view on their planned caesarean policy or rate

- Have a list of questions and note down answers as you may not remember details afterwards

- Clarify whether answers refer to hospital practice or reflect the opinion or preference of the practitioner you are speaking to

- Where relevant ask for references and follow them up

Hospital ratings

You may be able to access feedback about your hospital using patient opinion sites. Try keyword searches on the internet with phrases such as "patient review", "hospital ratings", "patient opinions". In the UK the following sites may be a good place to start: www.birthchoiceuk.com or www.patientopinion.org.uk. In the US www.healthgrades.com

---

Planning your birth

Questions to ask of your practitioners/hospital

Before labour

- What are the specific reasons suggesting I need a caesarean? Is this a recommendation or my only option?

- If only a recommendation, what is the likelihood of requiring an unplanned caesarean if I try for a vaginal delivery?

- What are the risks of this procedure for me and my baby?

- Can I let labour start before my caesarean?

- Can I still have a caesarean if I go into labour early?

- Is there a *cell saver* available (used in place of transfusions if you are at high risk of severe blood loss or cannot have a transfusion on religious grounds). This machine cleans and recycles your blood during surgery and is *not* widely available

- Can my baby stay with me throughout surgery assuming there are no complications?

- Can I breastfeed in theatre?

- Are there specialists to help me with breastfeeding once back on the ward?

- Can my partner stay with me during set-up and surgery?

- Can my partner stay with me outside visiting hours?

- Can I talk through my experience with someone who has been present at my birth?

- What specific practices vary from one team member to another?

- What are the financial costs to me of a caesarean and hospital recovery?

- Is there a Special Care Unit available? If not, where will my baby be sent for specialist care if it is needed?

- How many theatres are there?

- Are there private rooms available for after my birth? If so, how much are they and can I pre-book?

- These are my birth plan preferences, can you accommodate each of these?

- Confirm the hospital's policy on:
  - Timing (e.g. Can I wait till week 39? Can I wait to go into labour before surgery begins?)
  - Anaesthetic options (some hospitals do not offer combined anaesthetic)
  - Type of incision and closure technique
  - Post-operative pain medication options
  - VBAC
  - Intervention e.g. episiotomies, fetal monitoring
  - CDMR

- Where baby sleeps during my stay (it is rare to use nurseries but worth checking)
- Having a doula present as well as my partner
- Early discharge
- What are the hospital's statistics for:
  - Your specific condition (e.g. breech or multiple births)
  - Rates of medical interventions
  - VBAC (attempts and success)
- Clarify the hospital's approach to the caesarean procedure, including:
  - Pre-incision antibiotics
  - Vitamin K injections
  - Cord cut timing
  - Closure techniques
  - *Natural caesarean* procedures (see Chapter 1)

When in labour

- What are the specific reasons that mean I now need a caesarean?
- Is this still a recommendation or my only option? Are there any alternatives?
- A good question for gauging the severity of your situation is to ask - Is it safe to do nothing just yet?

Questions to ask your anaesthetist

- What anaesthetic options are most appropriate to my situation?
- What are the risks associated with this option for my baby and I?
- Is it safe to breastfeed immediately after this anaesthetic?

Questions to ask your doula/independent midwife

- What experience do they have? (If you have a specific condition or situation e.g. twins or breech, do they have experience of this?)
- What support can they offer during a caesarean?
- Have they had experience of my hospital?
- How can they guarantee their availability?

- How can they work with my birth partner?

- What are the fees and are there any hidden costs?

Planning a vaginal birth

There are lots of things to check if you are planning a vaginal delivery, from the facilities available if birthing in hospital, to the importance they place on timing of labour phases, policy on induction, pain relief and intervention rates and how they define *active* birth and so on. If you are hiring an independent midwife for a home birth the same applies, and you need to be particularly confident in their experience if you have specific conditions e.g. breech or twins etc.

Glossary

Adhesions – Scar tissue that forms after surgery. Sometimes this may attach two or more areas together (e.g. adhering the uterus to the bladder)

Anaesthetic – Pain relief drug used to remove sensation for a time

APGAR – The scoring mechanism used to define a baby's health. Scores are taken at 1 and 5 minutes after birth. A score of 8-10 reflects excellent condition, 5-7 fair condition and extra help may be needed, 5 or lower shows that your baby is in poor condition needing extra help. APGARs continue to be taken until she reaches an acceptable score

BMI (Body Mass Index) – A score that describes the relationship between your weight and height. A BMI over 25 is considered overweight

Breech – The position your baby is lying in - head up, bottom down

Caesarean – See Chapter 1 – Terminology

Catheter – Small tube used, in caesareans, to drain urine from the bladder

CDMR (Caesarean Delivery on Maternal Request) – A caesarean that has been requested by you. It has not originated from a practitioner's recommendation

Cephalic presentation – The ideal position that your baby will be lying in – head down

Cephalopelvic disproportion – Your baby's head is too large to fit through your pelvis

Cervix – The neck of the uterus

Classical incision – A vertical cut in the uterus. Rarely used and typically only with very premature or very large babies and those in a transverse position

Cord prolapse – Your baby's umbilical cord drops through the vagina risking compression and oxygen starvation prior to birth

Deep Vein Thrombosis (DVT) – A blood clot that forms in a deep vein

Diabetes – A medical condition where insufficient insulin is produced causing high blood sugar levels. This condition can begin during pregnancy and is referred to as gestational diabetes. Once diagnosed it is generally manageable but can cause your baby to be larger than average, increasing the likelihood of a caesarean

Dystocia – Medical term for true *failure to progress* i.e. the cervix has not continued (or in some cases even started) to open

Eclampsia – A severe form of pre-eclampsia including fitting and high blood pressure with a significant risk of blood clotting. A caesarean is required immediately

Electro-convulsive therapy (ECT) – Sometimes used to treat major depression, typically where other techniques have failed. It is also known as electric shock treatment

Electronic fetal monitoring – External electrodes monitor your baby's heartbeat while still in the womb

Endometritis – An inflammation of the uterus wall causing heavy bleeding and abdominal pain

Epidural – A type of regional anaesthetic used to numb a specific area, namely the abdomen. It can be used in both vaginal and caesarean births

Episiotomy – A surgical cut made in the perineum (between the vagina and anus) to ease the insertion of surgical instruments and/or to assist your baby's exit

Fetal blood sampling – This process can be used to determine how much oxygen is getting to your baby. A sample is taken usually from her head and is often in situations where practitioners are still trying to evaluate the need for a caesarean

Fetal distress – The medical term used to describe a baby that is becoming oxygen starved during delivery. If delivered immediately there should not be any long-term effects

Fetus – An unborn baby. Prior to 8 weeks gestation the baby is referred to as an embryo

Forceps – A medical instrument, operated in a pincer motion, used to clasp your baby's head to assist delivery. Their use sometimes requires an episiotomy

General anaesthetic – A type of anaesthesia used in situations where a fast delivery is essential or where regional anaesthetic is insufficient. It delivers a complete loss of both sensation and consciousness

Gestational age – The age of your baby, measured in weeks from the first day of your last period

Haemorrhage – An excessive loss of blood. It has different terms according to when the bleed occurs: antepartum – before birth, intrapartum – during birth, postpartum – after birth

Hysterectomy – A medical procedure to remove the cervix and uterus

Incontinence – A condition where you do not have full control of your bladder and/or bowel, often referred to as stress incontinence. Leakage occurs when coughing, laughing or sneezing

Induction – The use of artificial techniques to initiate labour. A *sweep* (the artificial separation of the membranes around your baby using a finger *sweeping* around the cervix) may be tried first and if this is unsuccessful then drugs (e.g. Syntocinon – a synthetic version of oxytocin) will be administered to try and trigger birth

Intravenous drip (IV) – A small tube inserted into the back of your hand through which additional fluids are administered, for example to rehydrate you during and after surgery or provide drugs to counteract expected drops in blood pressure

IVD – Instrumental Vaginal Delivery

Lochia – The normal blood and tissue lost through the vagina after any birth

Meconium – Often called *baby poo,* it is a by-product of your baby's growth while still in the womb. She may pass meconium during birth and this is sometimes viewed as a sign of her distress

Midwife – A person specially trained in the care of mothers and babies before, during and for up to 28 (UK) weeks after birth

Morbidity – The medical term for disease and illness, but not death

Mortality – The medical term for death

Obstetrician – A doctor specialising in pregnancy and birth (a gynaecologist specialises in women's health but not necessarily in pregnancy and birth)

Oxytocin – A hormone released during birth to make the uterus contract. It also stimulates the production of breast milk

Paediatrician – A doctor specialising in the care of infants, children and adolescents

PCA (Patient Controlled Anaesthetic) – A pain relief mechanism administered through the IV in the back of your hand whenever you press a button – up to a safe limit preset by the practitioner

Pelvic floor muscles – A group of muscles around the vagina and anus that supports the bladder and uterus

Perineum – The area of skin and muscle between the anus and vagina

Placenta – The organ that develops during pregnancy connecting your baby to you. Through the placenta and umbilical cord she will receive all the nutrients and oxygen she needs for growth

Prophylactic caesarean – A caesarean that is planned to ensure the safest outcome – in the mother's or the practitioner's opinion. In other words, an informed choice to specifically avoid certain outcomes e.g. to avoid HIV transmission or to avoid an instrumental vaginal birth

Regional anaesthetic – A type of anaesthesia affecting only part of the body. Epidurals and spinals are forms of regional anaesthetic

Respiratory difficulties – A condition your baby may experience, most commonly associated with premature birth. Respiratory problems for you are rare and typically associated with general anaesthetic (see Appendix C)

Scar dehiscence – The unintentional opening of an old scar. Dehiscence during pregnancy, if undetected and significant, can mean the membranes surrounding your baby rupture and expel your baby into the abdominal cavity, necessitating an immediate a caesarean

Shoulder dystocia – The failure of the shoulder to birth. In the very rare instances where this cannot be corrected a caesarean will be required

Special care unit (SCU) – A unit within many hospitals dedicated to the care of babies experiencing difficulties. Not all hospitals have such units and not all units will be able to accommodate all conditions, so in specific situations your baby may be transferred to another hospital

Spinal anaesthetic – A form of anaesthetic used to numb the abdomen and legs prior to a caesarean

Stillbirth – A baby that is born dead (any time after 23 gestational weeks)

SVD – Spontaneous vaginal delivery

Term – Commonly referred to as 40 weeks. However, a baby is considered to be *term* anywhere between 37 and 42 weeks and this varies slightly according to mother's ethnicity

Thrush – A fungal infection typically in the vaginal area but which can also occur on the nipples. On the nipples it can make breastfeeding very painful, you and your baby will need to be treated to prevent re-infection

Tokophobia – A severe dread of childbirth

Transverse position – Your baby is lying across your body rather than head up or down. If attempts to turn her are unsuccessful a caesarean will be necessary

Trial by scar or *Trial by labour* – A rather negative term used to classify those women aiming for a vaginal delivery after having a previous caesarean

Umbilical cord – The cord connecting your baby to the placenta. Through it she receives all the oxygen and nutrients (via the blood) that she needs to grow

Uterus – The organ in which your baby develops – also referred to as the womb

Vagina – The muscular canal that connects the uterus to the outside of your body

VBAC (Vaginal Birth After Caesarean) Where a homebirth is planned after a caesarean this may be noted as HVBAC

Ventouse – A suction cup that can be attached to your baby's head when she is having difficulties being born. Gripping her in this way enables her to be manoeuvred during contractions. This procedure is invasive and is sometimes accompanied by an episiotomy

Womb – The organ in which your baby develops, also referred to as the uterus

Other resources

Many of the resources below are UK based but offer email support wherever you are. Using these as starting points you should be able to track down similar organisations within your own country.

General birth resources

AIMS (Association for Improvement in Maternity Services) www.aims.org.uk A campaign group with lots of detailed information about birth issues, both vaginal and caesarean.

Babycentre.co.uk www.babycentre.co.uk A very detailed website covering most issues in an informed and sympathetic manner.

Birth Choice UK www.birthchoiceuk.com This resource helps you assess your maternity care options and provides up-to-date (UK) maternity statistics by location.

The Fat Ladies Club by H. Gardiner, A. Bettridge, S. Groves, A. Jones, L. Lawrence, Penguin Books (2002), ISBN-13: 978-0141007892. A down-to-earth look at five women's real experiences of pregnancy and childbirth.

The Girlfriend's Guide to Pregnancy by V. Iovine, Pocket Books (1995), ISBN-13: 978-0671524319. A realistic look at pregnancy and childbirth. Refreshingly honest about how you may feel and what you may experience physically and emotionally.

NCT (National Childbirth Trust) www.nctpregnancyandbabycare.com A charity and lobby group supporting families through pregnancy and beyond. Amongst other things they offer antenatal education and local groups to meet other mums.

What to Expect When You're Expecting by A. Eisenberg, H. Murkoff, S. Hathaway, Simon & Schuster Ltd (2002), ISBN-13: 978-1847373755. A weighty tome with information on pretty much everything you can think of.

Birth partners

Birth Trauma Association www.birthtraumaassociation.org.uk/fathers.htm Short stories from traumatised dads, how they coped and email addresses of two dads willing to offer support.

Dad.info www.dad.info Written by men for men, this is a good source of support on issues ranging from birth and family life to money, education and health.

Childdevelopmentinfo.com
www.childdevelopmentinfo.com/health_safety/birth_partner.shtml
A detailed article on the role of a birth partner.

Fatherhood by M. Berkmann, Vermillion (2005), ISBN-13: 978-0091900632.
A very detailed and humorous look at pregnancy, birth and fatherhood.

Fathers Direct www.fathersdirect.com A charity providing lots of information and support on all aspects of fatherhood.

Fathers Matter +44 1268 556328 email: alanwjenkins@btopenworld.com A recommendation from the Fatherhood Institute, this organisation has experience with postnatal depression in both men and women.

Midwivesonline.com
www.midwivesonline.com/parents/parents1/s_menu/245/baby/245/27 A midwife answers FAQs about being a birth partner.

My Wife's A Bitch! www.birthrites.org A short article giving a realistic insight into how it can feel when you partner gets pregnant.

Todaysparent.com
www.todaysparent.com/pregnancybirth/labour/article.jsp?content=6074&
page=1 A useful, detailed article on the role of a birth partner.

Birth professionals

Childbirth Connection
www.childbirthconnection.org/article.asp?ck=10146 A detailed list of American resources for finding birth centres and midwives.

Doula.com www.doula.com A clear information site describing the role of a doula and how to find one.

Doula UK www.doula.org.uk A charity offering excellent support in locating and defining the role of your doula.

Independent Midwives Association www.independentmidwives.org.uk FAQs relating to the role and potential of independent midwives. Also provides a means for locating (UK) independent midwives in your area. An excellent resource.

Royal College of Anaesthetists www.rcoa.ac.uk Detailed information about the benefits and risks of all forms of anaesthesia. It links to information specific to obstetric anaesthetics www.oaa-anaes.ac.uk/content.asp?ContentID=11 and is available in many languages.

RCOG (Royal College of Obstetricians and Gynaecologists) www.rcog.org.uk/womens-health/patient-information A useful site for checking the *official line* in obstetrics and gynaecology, with a detailed glossary of medical terms.

Birth trauma (PnD, PPnD and PTSD)

Association for Postnatal Illness (APNI) www.apni.org A charity providing information and counselling services to those suffering from, or those supporting those suffering from, postnatal depression. The free leaflets are excellent.

ASSIST www.traumatic-stress.freeserve.co.uk A charity offering support and practical advice to those experiencing trauma.

Birth Trauma Association (BTA) www.birthtraumaassociation.org.uk A charity and lobby group supporting women through traumatic birth experiences. There's also a useful article on understanding your medical notes and associated acronyms.

British Association for Behavioural and Cognitive Psychotherapies www.babcp.com A description of the therapy with the ability to search for a therapist in your area.

British Association of Counselling and Psychotherapy (BACP) www.bacp.co.uk/seeking_therapist/right_therapist.php Lots of advice on how to find a therapist to suit your needs, with a search facility. This is an international service despite being a UK association.

British Association of Psychotherapists www.bap-psychotherapy.org A detailed site describing treatment opportunities and a facility to locate a psychotherapist in your area.

Depression Alliance www.depressionalliance.org A detailed site offering advice, information and support.

Erbs Palsy www.erbspalsygroup.co.uk Raising awareness of and providing support to families affected by this medical condition that arises from nerve damage in the baby's neck.

European Fatherhood
www.european-fatherhood.com/UserFiles/File/Men%20and%20Postnatal%20Depression.pdf An interesting document for practitioners responsible for working with men suffering from postnatal depression. See preventative and treatment sections at the end particularly.

MAMA (Meet a Mum) www.mama.co.uk A charity providing information about postnatal depression and a means of putting mothers in touch with local groups whose aim is to provide friendship and support.

Postpartum men www.postpartummen.com/index.html A site full of information and ideas on dealing with male postnatal depression.

Breastfeeding

Association of Breastfeeding Mothers (ABM) www.abm.me.uk A charity offering helpline support and counselling to mothers experiencing difficulties.

Breastfeeding after a caesarean
www.plus-size-pregnancy.org/CSANDVBAC/bfaftercesarean.htm#Inhibition_of_Newborn_Suckling_Responses_by_Medications A detailed article about all aspects of breastfeeding following caesarean birth. Well researched and includes all references. Also talks about grieving breastfeeding.

The Breastfeeding Network (BfN) www.breastfeedingnetwork.org.uk A detailed information site with information on specific drugs and their safety.

La Leche www.laleche.org.uk or www.llli.org An international organisation offering breastfeeding support. The site contains excellent articles e.g. www.llli.org/llleaderweb/LV/LVAugSep00p63.html www.llli.org/FAQ/positioning.html

MOBI (Mothers Overcoming Breastfeeding Issues)
www.mobimotherhood.org/MM/default.aspx A support site for women coming to terms with unsuccessful breastfeeding. There are lots of articles and ideas.

Breastfeeding videos
www.breastfeeding.com/helpme/helpme_videos/video_informational.html
www.nhs.uk/Planners/pregnancycareplanner/pages/feedingbabyhome.aspx

Caesarean birth

Caesarean.org www.caesarean.org.uk Detailed site with book reviews, articles and useful personal stories.

Csections.org www.csections.org The author's website offering further commentary on the caesarean debate.

Electivecesarean.com www.electivecesarean.com An excellent site summarising the latest research on caesarean birth and offering online support.

Electivecesarean.com (blog) www.cesareandebate.blogspot.com An excellent insight into many aspects of the caesarean debate. It has clear information with lots of links to research.

NICE Caesarean Guideline
www.nice.org.uk/nicemedia/pdf/CG013NICEguideline.pdf
The UK guidelines for caesarean birth.

Photos of a caesarean birth in progress
www.fensende.com/Users/swnymph/csect/gallery.html
www.csectionrecovery.com

Video of a caesarean birth
www.mayoclinic.com/health/c-section/MM00531 A very detailed and
professional video of preparation and surgery.

Caesarean recovery (and general physical recovery)

Baby Centre www.babycentre.co.uk Articles tailored to caesarean recovery
and excellent forums for meeting women with similar experiences.

Caesarean Recovery by C. Gallegher-Mundy, Carrol and Brown (2006),
ISBN-13: 978-1904760429. An excellent book, two thirds about exercise,
diet and lifting guidance.

Csections Recovery www.csectionrecovery.com An excellent site with lots
of ideas and advice about recovery and a list of online forums.

Scar images www.caesarean.org.uk/ScarPics.html Graphic at times. These
are not professional photographs so the style and quality varies from one
image to the next.

Sex in Pregnancy and after Childbirth National Childbirth Trust
Brochure available from www.nctshop.co.uk/Get-Closer-Humps-and-
bumps/productinfo/1660

Death

Foundation for the Study of Infant Deaths www.fsid.org.uk An
organisation championing research in this area. Offers links to local
support people and an online forum.

M.I.S.S. Foundation www.misschildren.org/index.html Information,
support and links to local support groups for families experiencing the loss
of a child.

Stillbirths and Neonatal Death Society (SANDS) www.uk-sands.org A
charity and lobby group offering help and practical advice on what to do
and how to cope as bereaved parents.

Multiple birth

Twins and Multiple Birth Association (TAMBA) www.tamba.org.uk
Telephone and email support as well as local support groups around the
UK for families of twins. Also offers a short, practical course on coping with
the realities of multiple births.

The Multiple Births Foundation (MBF) www.multiplebirths.org.uk This organisation is aimed at both parents and professionals and concentrates on information and research.

Talk about Twins www.talk-about-twins.com/index.html An excellent site offering practical advice and information about coping with twins, not only through birth but as toddlers and throughout their school years.

Twinsclub.co.uk www.twinsclub.co.uk An online resource linking local twin clubs while providing forums and advice on parenting twins.

Parenthood

Secrets of the Baby Whisperer T. Hogg Ballatine Books (2005), ISBN-13: 9780345479099. An excellent resource during early parenting.

Cry-sis www.cry-sis.org.uk A charity offering support for families trying to cope with excessively crying, sleepless and demanding babies.

Fatherhood by M. Berkmann, Vermillion (2005), ISBN-13: 978-0091900632. A realistic look at parenthood specifically for dads.

The Incredible Years by C. Webster-Stratton, The Incredible Years (2006), ISBN-13: 978-1892222046. A troubleshooting guide to raising children.

Little Angels by T. Byron, S. Baveystock, BBC Books (2005), ISBN-13: 978-0563519416. An excellent, realistic parents guide to understanding your children.

Mumsnet www.mummumsnet.com Written by parents for parents. It has discussion groups and articles on many issues around parenting (as well as pregnancy and birth).

Netmums www.netmums.com This site offers connection to localised information for parents.

mums on babies by mumsnet.com, Cassell Illustrated (2003), ISBN-13: 978-1844030712. Parents' advice to other parents, gathered from the website www.mumsnet.com

One Sock, Three Shoes and No Hairbrush by R. Abrams, Cassell Illustrated (2001), ISBN-13: 978-0304354290. An excellent, realistic look at having your second child.

The Baby by J. Burningham Random House (1975), ISBN:13: 978-1564026897. A great book to use with your toddler to talk about the arrival of your new baby

There's going to be a baby by J. Burningham, Walker, (2010), ISBN-13: 978-0744549966. A great guide to the types of questions your toddler might ask and how to tackle them.

The Secret of Happy Children by S. Bidduiph, Thorsons (1998), ISBN-13: 978-0722536698. Explains how to listen to and with communicate with your children.

Three in a Bed: The Benefits of Sleeping with your Baby by D. Jackson, Bloomsbury Publishing PLC (2003), ISBN-13: 978-0747565758. A perspective on bed-sharing.

Special care

BLISS www.bliss.org.uk A charity and lobby group supporting families of premature babies, with local support groups (UK).

Life's Little Treasures Foundation www.lifeslittletreasures.org.au/?page_id=817 A charity supporting families of premature babies and children.

Turning your baby

Spinning Babies www.spinningbabies.com Information on how to help your baby turn into a better birth position.

Understanding and Teaching Optimal Fetal Positioning by J. Sutton and P. Scott, Birth Concepts (1996), ISBN-13: 978-0473041359. A practical introduction to this technique.

VBACS

Caesarean Birth and VBAC Information www.caesarean.org.uk Lots of information about VBACs. They also have a gallery of scar pictures.

How to Avoid an Unnecessary Caesarean by H. Churchill and W. Savage, Middlesex University Press (2008), ISBN-13: 978-1904750161. An informative, short read, covering the main issues.

Vaginal Birth After Caesarean: The VBAC Handbook by H. Churchill, W. Savage, Middlesex University Press (2008), ISBN-13: 978-1904750215. An informative, short read covering the main issues.

VBAC.co.uk www.vbac.co.uk Lots of VBAC stories.

Homebirth.org.uk www.homebirth.org.uk A detailed website covering all aspects of researching and planning a homebirth.

Vaginal births

Active Birth Centre www.activebirthcentre.com An organisation providing lots of information and classes on active birth, breastfeeding and recovery (UK).

Active Birth: The New Approach to Giving Birth Naturally by J. Balaskas, Harvard Common Press (1994), ISBN-13: 978-1558320383. All you need to know about active birthing.

Birthing from Within by P. England, R. Horowitz, Partera Press (1998), ISBN-13: 978-0285637870. Lots of information and techniques to assist you toward a natural birth goal. It includes pain management techniques, nutritional advice, art therapy and how to accommodate medical intervention.

Hypnobabies www.hypnobabies.com/ A complete course in self hypnosis for birth.

Ina May's Guide to Childbirth by I. Gaskin, Bantam Doubleday Dell (2003), ISBN-13: 978-0091924157. This book starts with powerful, positive birth stories, leading onto discussion of all aspects of natural childbirth. This is an excellent resource for those hoping to avoid medical intervention.

Vaginal birth plan templates

www.birthplan.com

www.nhs.uk/Planners/pregnancycareplanner/Pages/BirthPlan.aspx

Acknowledgements

I would have not been able to write this book without having first experienced the caesareans that delivered my two gorgeous girls. Their births were wonderful, truly inspiring and only a little scary.

A special thanks to my husband Simon who has had infinite patience with me and been a real link to sanity throughout my pregnancies and in the six years since.

Thanks too to all those people I interviewed, mums, dads and practitioners, who provided information and many more ideas about how to personalise, prepare for and recover from a caesarean, planned or otherwise.

Thanks to my parents Carol and Don who read the initial *huge* draft and all those who helped further refine it: Haley Cooper, Isabel Hogan, Linda Buxton, and those professionals who checked all the medical content. Thanks to my sister Alison whose enthusiasm for this project and faith in me has spurred me on and to Anne Ng whose idea it was to turn research for my own birth into a book to help others.

Professional contributors:

- Philip J Steer BSc, MD, RCOG Emeritus Professor, Imperial College London, Consultant Obstetrician, Chelsea and Westminster Hospital London

- Fiona Knox MB ChB, FRCA, MD – Consultant Anaesthetist

- Debbie Rhodes Registered Midwife RM (Hons) www.independentbirth.com

- Dr Lena M. Crichton, Consultant Obstetrician Aberdeen Maternity Hospital

- Dr Bryan Beattie MD FRCOG – Consultant in Fetal Medicine and Director of Innermost Secrets Ltd, Cardiff

- Dr Fiona Schneider FRCOG, Consultant Obstetrician and Gynaecologist

- Kim Hughes BSc (Hons) Registered Midwife RM www.yorkstorks.co.uk

- Maureen Treadwell – Co-founder of the Birth Trauma Association

- Penny Christensen – Executive Director Birth Trauma Canada

- Chris Warren – Registered Midwife RM www.yorkstorks.co.uk

- Christa Greenacre – NCT teacher (retired)

- Professor James Drife FRCOG

Thanks too to Catherine Lain for her wonderful editorial support in the final stages.

In addition to all the references already cited I used the following sources:

Books & Articles:

Caesarean birth in Britain: A Book for Health Professionals and Parents by C. Francome, W. Savage, H. Churchill, H. Lewison, Middlesex University Press, London (1993), ISBN: 13: 978-1898253006

Caesarean Birth – Your Questions Answered by D. Chippington Derrick, G. Lowdon, F. Barlow, NCT Publication (2004), ISBN-13: 978-0954301835

Cesarean section: Understanding and celebrating your baby's birth by M. Moore M, C. de Costa, John Hopkins University Press (2003), ISBN-13: 978-0801873379

The Essential C-section Guide by M. Connolly, D. Sullivan, Broadway Books (2004), ISBN-13: 978-0767916073

The Faceless Caesarean by C. Oblasser, BoD (2009) ISBN:13: 978-3837075601

Fatherhood Reclaimed by A. Burgess, Vermillion (1997) ISBN: 0 09 179020 4

How to Avoid an Unnecessary Caesarean by H. Churchill, W. Savage Middlesex University Press (2008) ISBN-13: 978-1904750161

Michael Odent's article on role of the father
www.midwiferytoday.com/articles/fatherpart.asp

Vaginal Birth After Caesarean by H. Churchill, W. Savage, Middlesex University Press (2008), ISBN-13: 978-1904750215

Websites:

About.com

AIMS.org.uk

Babycentre.co.uk

Baby-health.net

Birthrites.org

Birthtraumaassociation.org.uk

Caesarean.org.uk

Electivecesarean.com

NCTpregnancyandbabycare.com

Rcog.org.uk

References

1 NHS, *NHS Maternity Statistics 2008-9*, (NHS Information Centre, Dec 2009)

2 J. Thomas, S. Paranjothy and Royal College of Obstetricians and Gynaecologists Clinical Effectiveness Support Unit. *National sentinel caesarean section audit report*. (London: RCOG Press, 2001)

3 D.M. Haas, A.W. Ayres 'Laceration Injury at Cesarean Delivery' *Journal Maternal Fetal & Neonatal Medicine*, 11/3 (2002) 196-8

4 M. Connolly, D. Sullivan, *The Essential C-section Guide* (Broadway Books, 2004)

5 RCOG, *Birth After Previous Caesarean*, (RCOG, 2008)

6 J. Smith, F. Plaat, N. Fisk, 'The Natural Caesarean: a Woman-Centred Technique', *BJOG*, 115/8 (2008) 1037–1042

7 J. Moorhead 'Every bit as magical' *The Guardian*, 3rd December 2005

8 J. Smith, F. Plaat, N. Fisk, 'The Natural Caesarean: a Woman-Centred Technique', *BJOG*, 115/8 (2008) 1037–1042

9 NICE, *Guideline for Caesarean Section*, (National Institute for Clinical Excellence, 2004)

10 C. Francome, W. Savage, H. Churchill et al, *Caesarean Birth in Britain: A Book for Health Professionals and Parents* (London, Middlesex University Press, 1993)

11 NICE, *Guideline for Caesarean Section*, (National Institute for Clinical Excellence, 2004)

12 NHS, *Latest Maternity Statistics Show How the Pattern of Giving Birth in England is Changing*, (NHS Information Centre, 2008)

13 J. Oyston, 'A Guide to Spinal Anaesthesia for Caesarean Section for Anaesthetists and Anesthesiologists', www.uam.es [on-line article], 1996 - accessed March 2011 <http://www.uam.es/departamentos/medicina/anesnet/gtoa/cesarea/spinalcs.htm>

14 S. Paterson-Brown, 'Woman's Right – CS Following Patient's Request: Yes or No?' *The First World Congress On: Controversies in Obstetrics, Gynaecology & Infertility*, (Prague, 1999)

15 C. Oblasser, *The Faceless Caesarean* (BoD, 2009)

16 C. Francome, W. Savage, H. Churchill et al, *Caesarean Birth in Britain: A Book for Health Professionals and Parents* (London, Middlesex University Press, 1993)

17 NICE, *Guideline for Caesarean Section*, (National Institute for Clinical Excellence, 2004)

18 J.E. Soet, G.A. Brack, C. DiIorio, 'Prevalence and Predictors of Women's Experience of Psychological Trauma During Childbirth', *Birth*, 30 /1 (2003) 36-46

19 J. Lally, M. Murtagh, S. Macphail et al, 'More in Hope Than Expectation: A Systematic Review of Women's Expectations and Experience of Pain Relief in Labour' *BMC Medicine*, (2008) 6:7doi:10.1186/1741-7015-6-7

20 J. Lally, M. Murtagh, S. Macphail et al, 'More in Hope Than Expectation: A Systematic Review of Women's Expectations and Experience of Pain Relief in Labour' *BMC Medicine* (2008) 6:7doi:10.1186/1741-7015-6-7

21 NHS, *NHS Maternity Statistics 2008-9*, (NHS Information Centre, Dec 2009).

22 B.E. Hamilton, Martin J.A., S.J. Ventura, 'Births: Preliminary Data for 2007' *National Vital Statistics Report*, 57/12 (2009) 1-23

23 P. Roxby, 'Should there be a limit on caesareans?', *BBC Health News* [on-line article] June 2010 – accessed March 2011 <http://www.bbc.co.uk/news/10448034>

24 NHS, *Latest Maternity Statistics Show How the Pattern of Giving Birth in England is Changing*, (NHS Information Centre, 2008)

25 NHS, *NHS Maternity Statistics 2008-9*, (NHS Information Centre, Dec 2009).

26 Unknown, 'Birth in Britain Today Survey 2001', *Mother and Baby Magazine*, (2001)

27 E. Declercq, C. Sakala, M. Corry, et al, 'Listening to Mothers: Report of the First National U.S. Survey of Women's Childbearing Experiences' *Maternity Centre Association*, [on-line report], Oct. 2002 - accessed March 2011
< http://www.childbirthconnection.org/pdfs/LtMreport.pdf>

28 Birth Trauma Association, citing 'The Birth and Motherhood Survey' by Motherandbaby.com, (Conference notes, 2005)

29 Birth Trauma Association, citing 'The Birth and Motherhood Survey' by Motherandbaby.com, (Conference notes, 2005)

30 Birth Trauma Association, citing 'The Birth and Motherhood Survey' by Motherandbaby.com, (Conference notes, 2005)

31 Birth Trauma Association, citing 'The Birth and Motherhood Survey' by Motherandbaby.com, (Conference notes, 2005)

32 J. Thomas, S. Paranjothy and Royal College of Obstetricians and Gynaecologists Clinical Effectiveness Support Unit. *National sentinel caesarean section audit report*, (London: RCOG Press, 2001)

33 J. Chaney, 'Babble Talk: Do We Still Judge Women For Having C-Sections?' *Babble.com* [on-line article] April 2009 – accessed March 2011
<http://www.babble.com/CS/blogs/strollerderby/archive/2009/04/04/babble-talk-do-we-still-judge-women-for-having-c-sections.aspx>

34 J. Weaver, H. Statham, 'Wanting a caesarean section: the decision process' *BMJ*, 13/6 (2005) 1-5

35 A. Macfarlane, 'A question of delivery' *Healthmatters*, 46/15 (2001)

36 F. Bragg, D.A. Cromwell, L.C. Edozien et al, 'Variation in rates of caesarean section among English NHS trusts after accounting for maternal and clinical risk: cross sectional study' *BMJ*, (2010) 341, c5065

37 M. Viswanathan, A.G. Visco, K. Hartmann et al, 'Cesarean Delivery on Maternal Request. Evidence Report/Technology Assessment No. 133' *RTI International-University of North Carolina Evidence-Based Practice Center* under Contract No. 290-02-0016.) AHRQ Publication No. 06-E009 (2006)

38 NIH 'NIH State-of-the-Science Conference Statement on Cesarean Delivery on Maternal Request' *NIH Consensus State of the Science Statements*, 23/1 (2006) 1–29

39 J. Svigos, 'Commentary on 'Maternal Outcomes Associated with Planned Vaginal Versus Planned Primary Cesarean Delivery. F1000: "Changes Clinical Practice"' *Medscape Today* [on-line article] April 2010 – accessed April 2010 < http://www.medscape.com/medscapetoday>

40 K. Kallen, P.O. Olausson, 'Neonatal Mortality for Low-Risk Women by Method of Delivery' Letters in *BIRTH,* 34/1 (2007) 99-100

41 M. Connolly, D. Sullivan, *The Essential C-section Guide,* (Broadway Books, 2004)

42 J. Weaver, H. Statham, 'Wanting a caesarean section: the decision process' *BMJ,* 13/6 (2005) 1-5

43 NICE, *Guideline for Caesarean Section,* (National Institute for Clinical Excellence, 2004)

44 GMC *Priorities and Choices: Guidance from the General Medical Council* (GMC, 2000)

45 NICE, *Guideline for Caesarean Section,* (National Institute for Clinical Excellence, 2004)

46   GMC, *Consent Guidance: Patients and Doctors Making Decisions Together,* (General Medical Council, 2008)

47 NICE, *Guideline for Caesarean Section,* (National Institute for Clinical Excellence, 2004)

48 GMC, *Consent Guidance: Patients and Doctors Making Decisions Together,* (General Medical Council, 2008)

49 NICE, *Guideline for Caesarean Section,* (National Institute for Clinical Excellence, 2004)

50 NICE, *Guideline for Caesarean Section,* (National Institute for Clinical Excellence, 2004)

51 GMC, *Consent Guidance: Patients and Doctors Making Decisions Together,* (General Medical Council, 2008)

52 Birth Trauma Association, citing E. Kant, 'Childbirth and Human Rights' (Conference notes, 2005)

53 S. Paterson-Brown, 'Should Doctors Perform an Elective Caesarean Section on Request?' *BMJ,* 317 (1998) 462

54 Childbirthconnections.org 'Cascade of Intervention in Childbirth' *Childbirth Connection* [on-line article] u.d. - accessed March 2010 <www.childbirthconnection.org/ article.asp?ck=10182>

55 L. Penna, 'Caesarean Section on Request for Non-medical Indications' *Current Obstetric and Gynaecology,* 14 (2004) 22-223

56 K. Bole, 'Patience During Stalled Labor can Avoid C-sections' *University of California* [Press release] Oct 2008- accessed March 2011 <http://www.ucsf.edu/news/2008/10/4158/patience-during-stalled-labor-can-avoid-many-c-sections-ucsf-study-shows>

57 Z. Alfirevic, D. Devane, G.M.L. Gyte 'Continuous cardiotocography (CTG) as a Form of Electronic Fetal Monitoring (EFM) for Fetal Assessment During Labour' *Cochrane Database of Systematic Reviews 3.* Art. No.: CD006066. DOI: 10.1002/14651858.CD006066 (2006)

58 NICE, *Guideline for Caesarean Section,* (National Institute for Clinical Excellence, 2004)

59 M. Connolly, D. Sullivan, *The Essential C-section Guide,* (Broadway Books, 2004)

60 J. Lally, M. Murtagh, S. Macphail et al, 'More in Hope Than Expectation: A Systematic Review of Women's Expectations and Experience of Pain Relief in Labour' *BMC Medicine,* (2008) 6:7doi:10.1186/1741-7015-6-7

61 Z. Alfirevic, D. Devane, G.M.L. Gyte 'Continuous cardiotocography (CTG) as a Form of Electronic Fetal Monitoring (EFM) for Fetal Assessment During Labour' *Cochrane Database of Systematic Reviews 3.* Art. No.: CD006066. DOI: 10.1002/14651858.CD006066 (2006)

62 NICE, *Guideline for Caesarean Section*, (National Institute for Clinical Excellence, 2004)

63 NICE, *Guideline for Intrapartum Care,* (National Institute for Clinical Excellence, 2007)

64 J. Zhang, M.K. Yancey, M.A. Klebanoff et al, 'Does Epidural Analgesia Prolong Labor and Increase Risk of Cesarean Delivery? A Natural Experiment' *American Journal of Obstetrics & Gynaecology,* 185/1 (2001) 128-34

65 H. Churchill, W. Savage, *Vaginal Birth After Caesarean,* (Middlesex University Press, 2008)

66 J. Zhang, M.K. Yancey, M.A. Klebanoff et al, 'Does Epidural Analgesia Prolong Labor and Increase Risk of Cesarean Delivery? A Natural Experiment' *American Journal of Obstetrics & Gynecology,* 185/1 (2001) 128-34

67 S.L Eriksson, P.O. Olausson, C. Olofson, 'Use of Epidural Analgesia and its Relation to Caesarean and Instrumental Deliveries: A Population Based Study of 94,217 Primiparae' *European Journal of Obstetrics & Gynecology & Reproductive Biology,* 128/1-2 (2006) 270-5

68 C.A. Wong, B.M Scavone, A. M. Peaceman et al 'The Risk of Cesarean Delivery with Neuraxial Analgesia Given Early versus Late in Labor' *New England Journal of Medicine,* 352/7 (2005) 655-665

69 NICE, *Guideline for Intrapartum Care,* (National Institute for Clinical Excellence, 2007)

70 M. Enkin, M. Keirse, J. Neilson et al *A Guide to Effective Care in Pregnancy and Childbirth,* (Oxford University Press, 2000), Chapter 29 - 'Hospital Practices'

71 ICAN 'How to Avoid an Unnecessary Caesarean' *Childbirth.org* [on-line article] 1992 - accessed March 2011 <http://www.childbirth.org/section/avoid.html>

72 NICE, *Guideline for Caesarean Section*, (National Institute for Clinical Excellence, 2004)

73 M. Singata, J. Tranmer, G.M.L. Gyte, 'Restricting Oral Fluid and Food Intake During Labor' *Cochrane Database of Systematic Reviews* Issue 1. Art. No.: CD003930. DOI: 10.1002/14651858.CD003930.pub2 (2010)

74 M. Kubli, M.J. Scrutton, P.T. See et al 'An Evaluation of Isotonic Sports Drinks During Labor' *Anesthesia & Analgesia,* 94/2 (2002) 404-408

75 Churchill H Savage W, *How to Avoid an Unnecessary Caesarean,* (Middlesex University Press, 2008)

76 E.D. Hodnett, S. Gates, G.J. Hofmeyr et al 'Continuous Support for Women During Childbirth' *Cochrane Database of Systematic Reviews,* Issue 3. Art. No.: CD003766. DOI: 10.1002/14651858.CD003766.pub2 (2007)

77 J. Thomas, S. Paranjothy and Royal College of Obstetricians and Gynaecologists Clinical Effectiveness Support Unit. *National sentinel caesarean section audit report,* (London: RCOG Press, 2001)

78 M. Enkin, M. Keirse, J. Neilson et al *A Guide to Effective Care in Pregnancy and Childbirth,* (Oxford University Press, 2000), Chapter 28 - 'Social and Professional Support in Childbirth

79 E.D. Hodnett, S. Gates, G.J. Hofmeyr et al 'Continuous Support for Women During Childbirth' *Cochrane Database of Systematic Reviews,* Issue 3. Art. No.: CD003766. DOI: 10.1002/14651858.CD003766.pub2 (2007)

80 S. Guendelman, M. Pearl, S. Graham et al, 'Maternity Leave in the Ninth Month of Pregnancy and Birth Outcomes Among Working Women' *Women's Health Issues,* 19/1 (2009) 30-7

81 A. M. Cyna, G.L. McAuliffe, M.I Andrew, 'Hypnosis for Pain Relief in Labour and Childbirth: A Systematic Review' *British Journal of Anaesthesia*, 93/4 (2004) 505-11

82 A. Martin, P. Schauble, S. Raj et al 'Effects of Hypnosis on the Labor Processes and Birth Outcomes of Pregnant Adolescents' *Journal of Family Practice*, May Edition (2001)

83 M. B. Landon, S. Leindecker, C. Y. Spong et al 'The MFMU Cesarean Registry: Factors Affecting the Success of Trial of Labor After Previous Cesarean Delivery' *American Journal of Obstetrics & Gynecology*, 193/3 (2005) 1016-23

84 C. Gyamfi, G. Juhasz, P. Gyamfi et al 'Increased Success of Trial of Labor After Previous Vaginal Birth After Cesarean' *Obstetrics & Gynecology* 104/4 (2004) 715-9

85 H. Churchill, W. Savage, *Vaginal Birth After Caesarean*, (Middlesex University Press, 2008)

86 S. Tahseen, M. Griffiths, 'Vaginal Birth After Two Caesarean Sections (VBAC-2)— A Systematic Review with Meta-analysis of Success Rate and Adverse Outcomes of VBAC-2 Versus VBAC-1 and Repeat (third) Caesarean Sections' *BJOG*, 117/1 (2009)

87 RCOG, *Birth After Previous Caesarean*, (RCOG, 2008)

88 H. Churchill, W. Savage, *Vaginal Birth After Caesarean*, (Middlesex University Press, 2008)

89 A. G. Cahill, M. Tuuli, A. Odibo et al, 'Vaginal Birth After Caesarean for Women with Three or More Prior Caesareans: Assessing Safety and Success' *BJOG*, 117/4 (2010) 422-427

90 Childbirthconnections.org 'Caesarean Section - Why does the National US Cesarean Section rate keep going up?' *Childbirthconnections.org* [on-line article] Oct 2010 - accessed March 2011
<http://www.childbirthconnection.org/article.asp?ck=10456>

91 G. Lowdon, D. Chippington Derrick, 'VBAC - On Whose terms?' *AIMS Journal* 14/1 (2002)

92 RCOG, *Birth After Previous Caesarean*, (RCOG, 2008)

93 RCOG, *Birth After Previous Caesarean*, (RCOG, 2008)

94 RCOG, *Birth After Previous Caesarean*, (RCOG, 2008)

95 M. J. McMahon, E. R. Luther, W. A. Bowes et al 'Comparison of a Trial of Labor with an Elective Second Cesarean Section' *New England Journal of Medicine*, 335 (1996) 689-95

96 RCOG, *Birth After Previous Caesarean*, (RCOG, 2008)

97 H. Churchill, W. Savage, *Vaginal Birth After Caesarean* (Middlesex University Press, 2008)

98 RCOG, *Birth After Previous Caesarean*, (RCOG, 2008)

99 NICE, *Guideline for Caesarean Section*, (National Institute for Clinical Excellence, 2004)

100 RCOG, *Birth After Previous Caesarean*, (RCOG, 2008)

101 RCOG, *Birth After Previous Caesarean*, (RCOG, 2008)

102 M. Treadwell, 'Women Choosing Caesarean Have Low Death Rate' *Birth Trauma Association*, [Press release] Oct 2008

103 CEMACH, 'Saving Mothers Lives - 2003-2005' *Confidential Enquiry into Maternal and Child Health*, (2007) The Seventh Report of the Confidential Enquiries into Maternal Deaths in the United Kingdom

104 S. Fenwick, J. Alexander, 'Achieving Normality: The Key to Status Passage to Motherhood After a Caesarean Section' *Midwifery*, 25/5 (2009) 554-563

105 J. Lally, M. Murtagh, S. Macphail et al, 'More in Hope Than Expectation: A Systematic Review of Women's Expectations and Experience of Pain Relief in Labour' *BMC Medicine*, (2008) 6:7doi:10.1186/1741-7015-6-7

106 M. Moore, C. de Costa, *Cesarean Section: Understanding and Celebrating Your Baby's Birth*, (John Hopkins University Press, 2003)

107 K. Cox, J.D. Schwartz, *The Well-informed Patient's Guide to Caesarean Births*, (Dell Pub Co; Reissue edition, 1991)

108 M. Enkin, M. Keirse, J. Neilson et al *A Guide to Effective Care in Pregnancy and Childbirth* (Oxford University Press, 2000), Chapter 43 - 'Prophylactic Antibiotics with Cesarean Section'

109 F. Smaill, G.J. Hofmeyr, 'Antibiotic prophylaxis for cesarean section' *Cochrane Database of Systematic Reviews* Issue 3. Art. No.:CD000933. DOI:10.1002/14651858.CD000933 (2002)

110 Science Daily 'Delayed Umbilical Cord Clamping Boosts Iron In Infants' *Sciencedaily.com* [on-line article] 2006 - accessed March 2011

111 J. Mercer, D. Erickson-Owens, 'Delayed Cord Clamping Increases Infants' Iron Stores' *Lancet*, 367 (2006) 1956-7

112 NICE, *Guideline for Caesarean Section*, (National Institute for Clinical Excellence, 2004)

113 I. Gaertner, T. Burkhardt, E. Beinder, 'Scar Appearance of Different Skin and Subcutaneous Tissue Closure Techniques in Caesarean Section: A Randomized Study' *European Journal of Obstetrics, Gynecology and Reproductive Bio*logy, 138/1 (2008) 29-33

114 A. Cromi, F. Ghezzi, A. Gottardi, 'Cosmetic Outcomes of Various Skin Closure Methods Following Cesarean Delivery: A Randomized Trial' *American Journal of Obstetrics & Gynecology*, 203/1 2010) 36

115 K. Hofberg, M. R. Ward, 'Fear Of Pregnancy And Childbirth' *Postgraduate Medical Journal*, 79 (2003) 505-510

116 J. Lally, M. Murtagh, S. Macphail et al, 'More in Hope Than Expectation: A Systematic Review of Women's Expectations and Experience of Pain Relief in Labour' *BMC Medicine*, (2008) 6:7doi:10.1186/1741-7015-6-7

117 J. Lally, M. Murtagh, S. Macphail et al, 'More in Hope Than Expectation: A Systematic Review of Women's Expectations and Experience of Pain Relief in Labour' *BMC Medicine*, (2008) 6:7doi:10.1186/1741-7015-6-7

118 B.H. McCrea, M. E. Wright, 'Satisfaction In Childbirth And Perceptions Of Personal Control In Pain Relief During Labour' *Journal of Advanced Nursing*, 29/4 (1999) 877-884

119 J. Green, H. Baston, S. Easton, 'Greater Expectations? Inter-Relationships Between Women's Expectations And Experiences of Decision Making, Continuity, Choice and Control in Labour, and Psychological Outcomes: Summary Report' *Leeds: Mother & Infant Research Unit*, (2003)

120 NHS, *Latest Maternity Statistics Show How the Pattern of Giving Birth in England is Changing*, (NHS Information Centre, 2008)

121 B.E. Hamilton, Martin J.A., S.J. Ventura, 'Births: Preliminary Data for 2007' *National Vital Statistics Report*, 57/12 (2009) 1-23

122 J. Green, H. Baston, S. Easton, 'Greater Expectations? Inter-Relationships Between Women's Expectations And Experiences of Decision Making, Continuity, Choice and Control in Labour, and Psychological Outcomes: Summary Report' *Leeds: Mother & Infant Research Unit*, (2003)

123 J. Green, H. Baston, S. Easton, 'Greater Expectations? Inter-Relationships Between Women's Expectations And Experiences of Decision Making, Continuity, Choice and Control in Labour, and Psychological Outcomes: Summary Report' *Leeds: Mother & Infant Research Unit,* (2003)

124 NHS, *Latest Maternity Statistics Show How the Pattern of Giving Birth in England is Changing,* (NHS Information Centre, 2008)

125 J. Robinson, 'Psychological birth trauma' 2003 *AIMS Journal*,15/3 (2003)

126 Y. Hauck, J. Fenwick, J. Downie et al 'The Influence of Childbirth Expectations on Western Australian Women's Perceptions of Their Birth Experience' *Midwifery*, 23/3 (2007) 235-7

127 J. Lally, M. Murtagh, S. Macphail et al, 'More in Hope Than Expectation: A Systematic Review of Women's Expectations and Experience of Pain Relief in Labour' *BMC Medicine,* (2008) 6:7doi:10.1186/1741-7015-6-7

128 D. Murphy, C. Pope, J. Frost et al, 'Women's Views on the Impact of Operative Delivery in the Second Stage of Labour: Qualitative Interview Study' *BMJ,* 327 (2003) 1132

129 T. Mirvis, 'In Praise of the C-Section' *Babble.com* [on-line article] March 2009 – accessed March 2011 <http://www.babble.com/pregnancy/giving-birth/Im-not-sorry-I-didnt-have-a-natural-birth-In-Praise-of-the-C-Section/>

130 M. Connolly, D. Sullivan, *The Essential C-section Guide,* (Broadway Books, 2004)

131 E. R. Moore, G. C. Anderson, N. Bergman 'Early Skin-to-skin Contact for Mothers and their Healthy Newborn Infants' *Journal of Advanced Nursing,* 6/4 (2008) 439-40

132 K. Bolling, C. Grant, B. Hamlyn et al, 'Infant Feeding Survey 2005' *(NHS The Information Centre National Statistics,* 2007)

133 K.G. Dewey, 'Maternal and Fetal Stress Are Associated with Impaired Lactogenesis in Humans' *Journal of Nutrition,* 131 (2001) 3012-3015

134 R. Grajeda, R. Pérez-Escamilla. 'Stress During Labor and Delivery Is Associated with Delayed Onset of Lactation among Urban Guatemalan Women '*Journal of Nutrition,* 132 (2002) 3055-60

135 C. Tatano Beck, S. Watson, 'Impact of Birth Trauma on Breastfeeding: A Tale of Two Pathways' *Nursing Research,* 57/4 (2007) 228-236

136 Kmom 'Breastfeeding After A Cesarean' *Kmom* (2002 – accessed March 2011) <http://www.plus-size-pregnancy.org/CSANDVBAC/bfaftercesarean.htm>

137 G. Agboado, E. Michel, E. Jackson et al, 'Factors Associated with Breastfeeding Cessation in Nursing Mothers in a Peer Support Programme in Eastern Lancashire' *BMC Pediatrics* 10/3 (2010)

138 Birth Trauma Association, citing 'The Birth and Motherhood Survey' by Motherandbaby.com, (Conference notes, 2005)

139 Birth Trauma Association, citing 'The Birth and Motherhood Survey' by Motherandbaby.com, (Conference notes, 2005)

140 G. Barrett, J. Peacock, I Manyonda, 'Caesareans: a Short-Lived Honeymoon, Says Study into Sexual Function' *Brunel University and St George's Healthcare NHS Trust Press Release,* (2006)

141 M. Connolly, D. Sullivan, *The Essential C-section Guide* (Broadway Books, 2004)

142 E.L. Ryding, K. Wijma, B. Wijma, 'Psychological Impact of Emergency Cesarean Section in Comparison with Elective Cesarean Section, Instrumental and Normal Vaginal Delivery' *Journal of Psychosomatic Obstetrics & Gynecology* 19/3 (1998) 135-44

143 D. Murphy, C. Pope, J. Frost et al, 'Women's Views on the Impact of Operative Delivery in the Second Stage of Labour: Qualitative Interview Study' *BMJ,* 327 (2003) 1132

144 Y. Hauck, J. Fenwick, J. Downie et al 'The Influence of Childbirth Expectations on Western Australian Women's Perceptions of Their Birth Experience' *Midwifery,* 23/3 (2007) 235-7

145 J. Fisher, J. Astbury, A. Smith, 'Adverse Psychological Impact of Operative Obstetric Interventions: A Prospective Study' *Australian and New Zealand Journal of Psychiatry* 31/5 (1997) 728-738

146 C. Francome, W. Savage, H. Churchill et al, *Caesarean Birth in Britain: A Book for Health Professionals and Parents* (London, Middlesex University Press, 1993)

147 D. Murphy, C. Pope, J. Frost et al, 'Women's Views on the Impact of Operative Delivery in the Second Stage of Labour: Qualitative Interview Study' *BMJ,* 327 (2003) 1132

148 T. Solantaus, S. Salo, 'Paternal Postnatal Depression: Fathers Emerge from the Wings' *Lancet,* 365/9478 (2005) 2158-9

149 UK Men's Movement www.ukmm.org.uk – accessed March 2010

150 A. Burgess, *Fatherhood Reclaimed* (Vermillion, 1997)

151 R. Fletcher, S. Silberberg, D. Galloway, 'New Fathers' Postbirth Views of Antenatal Classes: Satisfaction, Benefits, and Knowledge of Family Services' *Journal of Perinatal Education,* 13/3 (2004) 18–26

152 M. Berkmann, *Fatherhood* (Vermillion, 2005)

153 A. Burgess A 'Maternal and Infant Health in the Perinatal Period: The Father's Role Literature Review' *Fatherhood Institute,* [on-line article] April 2008 – accessed March 2010, <http://www.fatherhoodinstitute.org/uploads/publications/356.pdf>

154 A. Burgess A 'Maternal and Infant Health in the Perinatal Period: The Father's Role Literature Review' *Fatherhood Institute,* [on-line article] April 2008 – accessed March 2010, <http://www.fatherhoodinstitute.org/uploads/publications/356.pdf>

155 A. Burgess A 'Maternal and Infant Health in the Perinatal Period: The Father's Role Literature Review' *Fatherhood Institute,* [on-line article] April 2008 – accessed March 2010, <http://www.fatherhoodinstitute.org/uploads/publications/356.pdf>

156 K. Erlandsson, A. Dsilna, I. Fagerberg et al 'Skin-to-skin Care with the Father after Cesarean Birth and its Effect on Newborn Crying and Prefeeding Behavior' *Birth* 34/2 (2007) 105-14

157 A. Burgess A 'Maternal and Infant Health in the Perinatal Period: The Father's Role Literature Review' *Fatherhood Institute,* [on-line article] April 2008 – accessed March 2010, <http://www.fatherhoodinstitute.org/uploads/publications/356.pdf>

158 A. Burgess, *Fatherhood Reclaimed* (Vermillion, 1997)

159 Working with Men Group 'Antenatal care and expectant fathers' 2007

160 PANDA (Post and Antenatal Depression Association) 'Men and Postnatal Depression: How Postnatal Depression can Affect Fathers' *Raising Children Network* [on-line article] Jan. 2010 - accessed March 2010
<http://raisingchildren.net.au/articles/men_and_postnatal_depression.html>

161 K. Deater-Deckard, K. Pickering, J.F. Dunn et al, 'Family Structure and Depressive Symptoms in Men Preceding and Following the Birth of a Child' *American Journal of Psychiatry* 155 (1998) 818-823

162 A. Burgess, *Fatherhood Reclaimed* (Vermillion, 1997)

163 A. Burgess A 'Maternal and Infant Health in the Perinatal Period: The Father's Role Literature Review' *Fatherhood Institute*, [on-line article] April 2008 – accessed March 2010, <http://www.fatherhoodinstitute.org/uploads/publications/356.pdf>

164 M. Berkmann, *Fatherhood* (Vermillion, 2005)

165 M. Berkmann, *Fatherhood* (Vermillion, 2005)

166 A. Burgess, *Fatherhood Reclaimed* (Vermillion, 1997)

167 *Biology of Dads* (2010) BBC TV Production

168 FatherFacts,'Father Facts: What good are Dads?' *FathersDirect.com*, 1/1 (2001)

169 M. Moore, C. de Costa, *Cesarean Section: Understanding and Celebrating Your Baby's Birth* (John Hopkins University Press, 2003)

170 S.J. Davey, S. Dziurawiec, A. O'Brien-Malone, 'Men's Voices: Postnatal Depression From the Perspective of Male Partners' *Qualitative Health Research*, 16/2 (2006) 206-220

171 C. Huang, L. Warner, 'Relationship Characteristics & Depression Among Fathers with Newborns' *Social Service Review* 79, (2005) 95-118

172 Fatherhood Institute, 'Fathers and Postnatal Depression: Research Results from the Project: Men's Psychological Transition to Fatherhood – Mood Disorders in Men Becoming Fathers' *Fatherhood Institute*, [on-line article] Aug 2010 – accessed Sept. 2010 < http://www.fatherhoodinstitute.org/2010/fatherhood-institute-research-summary-fathers-and-postnatal-depression/>

173 Surviving Depression 'Male Depression' *Surviving* Depression accessed Aug. 2010 <http://www.survivingdepression.net/types/male.html>

174 J. Milgrom, P. Mccloud, 'Parenting stress and postnatal depression' *Stress Medicine*, 12 (1996) 177–186

175 NICE, *Guideline for Caesarean Section*, (National Institute for Clinical Excellence, 2004)

176 B. Beattie, (Innermost Secrets Ltd, Aug 2010)

177 R.E. Davis-Floyd 'The Technocratic Body: American Childbirth as Cultural Expression' *Social Science & Medicine* 38/8 (1994) 1125-1140

178 NICE, *Guideline for Caesarean Section*, (National Institute for Clinical Excellence, 2004)

179 NICE, *Guideline for Caesarean Section*, (National Institute for Clinical Excellence, 2004)

180 P. Ko, Y. Yoon, 'Placenta Previa' *Emedicine.medscape.com* [on-line article] Aug 2009 – accessed Aug 2010 < http://emedicine.medscape.com/article/796182-overview>

181 RCOG *Placenta Praevia and Placenta Praevia Accreta: Diagnosis and Management* (RCOG, 2005)

182 A.T. Papageorghiou, C.K. Yu, I.E. Erasmus et al, 'Assessment of Risk for the Development of Pre-eclampsia by Maternal Characteristics and Uterine Artery Doppler', *BJOG*, 112 (2005) 703-9

183 L.C. Poon, V. Stratieva, S. Piras et al, 'Hypertensive Disorders in Pregnancy: Combined Screening by Uterine Artery Doppler, Blood Pressure and Serum PAPP-A at 11-13 weeks' *Prenatal.Diagnosis,* 30 (2010) 216-23

184 NICE, *Guideline for Caesarean Section,* (National Institute for Clinical Excellence, 2004)

185 RCOG *Management of genital herpes in pregnancy,* (RCOG, 2007)

186 RCOG *Umbilical Cord Prolapse in Late Pregnancy - Information For You* (RCOG, 2009)

187 RCOG *A Breech Baby at the End of Pregnancy - Information For You,* (RCOG, 2008)

188 M.E. Hannah, W.J. Hannah, S.A. Hewson et al, 'Planned Caesarean Section Versus Planned Vaginal Birth for Breech Presentation at Term: A Randomised Multicentre Trial' *Lancet* 356/9239 (2000)1375-83

189 A. M. Gülmezoglu, C.A. Crowther, P. Middleton, 'Induction of Labor for Improving Birth Outcomes for Women at or Beyond Term' *Cochrane Database of Systematic Reviews* Issue 4. Art. No.: CD004945. DOI: 10.1002/14651858.CD004945.pub2 (2006)

190 Childbirthconnections.org 'Cascade of Intervention in Childbirth' *Childbirth Connection* [on-line article] u.d. - accessed March 2010 <www.childbirthconnection.org/ article.asp?ck=10182>

191 J. Thomas, S. Paranjothy and Royal College of Obstetricians and Gynaecologists Clinical Effectiveness Support Unit. *National sentinel caesarean section audit report.* (London: RCOG Press, 2001)

192 NICE, *Guideline for Caesarean Section,* (National Institute for Clinical Excellence, 2004)

193 NICE, *Guideline for Caesarean Section,* (National Institute for Clinical Excellence, 2004)

194 T.J. Garite, R.H. Clark, J. P. Elliott et al, 'Twins and Triplets: The Effect of Plurality and Growth on Neonatal Outcome Compared with Singleton Infants' *American Journal of Obstetrics and Gynecology* 191/3 (2004) 700-707

195 G.C.S. Smith, J.P. Pell, R. Dobbie, 'Birth Order, Gestational Age, and Risk of Delivery Related Perinatal Death in Twins: Retrospective Cohort Study' *BMJ* 325 (2002) 1004-6

196 C. Spencer, D. Murphy, S. Bewley, 'Caesarean Delivery in the Second Stage of Labor: Better Training in Instrumental Delivery May Reduce Rates' *BMJ* 333/7569 (2006) 613-61

197 Y.B. Cheung, P. Yip, J. Karlberg, 'Mortality of Twins and Singletons by Gestational Age: A Varying-Coefficient Approach' *American Journal of Epidemiology* 152/12 (2000) 1107-1116

198 G.C.S. Smith, J.P. Pell, R. Dobbie, 'Birth Order, Gestational Age, and Risk of Delivery Related Perinatal Death in Twins: Retrospective Cohort Study' *BMJ* 325 (2002) 1004-6

199 M. Enkin, M. Keirse, J. Neilson et al *A Guide to Effective Care in Pregnancy and Childbirth* (Oxford University Press, 2000), Chapter 31 - 'Monitoring the Progress of Labor'

200 J. Thomas, S. Paranjothy and Royal College of Obstetricians and Gynaecologists Clinical Effectiveness Support Unit. *National sentinel caesarean section audit report.* (London: RCOG Press, 2001)

201 A.N. Rosenthal, S. Paterson-Brown, 'Is There an Incremental Rise in the Risk of Obstetric Intervention with Increasing Maternal Age?' *British Journal of Obstetrics & Gynaecology,* 105/10 (1998) 1064-9

202 A.N. Rosenthal, S. Paterson-Brown, 'Is There an Incremental Rise in the Risk of Obstetric Intervention with Increasing Maternal Age?' *British Journal of Obstetrics & Gynaecology,* 105/10 (1998) 1064-9

203 G. S. Berkowitz, M.L. Skovron, R.H. Lapinski et al 'Delayed Childbearing and the Outcome of Pregnancy' *New England Journal of Medicine*, 322 (1990) 659-664

204 H.A. Al-Turki, A. T. Abu-Heija, M.H. Al-Sibai, 'The Outcome of Pregnancy in Elderly Primigravidas' *Saudi Medical Journal*, 11 (2003) 1230-3

205 J. S. Bell, D.M Campbell, W. J. Graham et al, 'Do Obstetric Complications Explain High Caesarean Section Rates Among Women Over 30? A Retrospective Analysis' *BMJ* (2001) 322 : 894 doi: 10.1136/bmj.322.7291.894

206 A. Rosenthal, 'Maternal Age is Important' *BMJ* 318/7176 (1999) 120 – Response 6

207 A. Rosenthal, 'Maternal Age is Important' *BMJ* 318/7176 (1999) 120 – Response 6

208 J. Weaver, 'Complications, or Fear of Complications? A Rapid Response to Bell JS et al' - 'Do Obstetric Complications Explain High Caesarean Section Rates Among Women Over 30? A Retrospective Analysis' (2001) *BMJ* 322:894 doi:10.1136/bmj.322.7291.894

209 D. Rajasingam, P. T. Seed, A. L Briley et al, 'A Prospective Study of Pregnancy Outcome and Biomarkers of Oxidative Stress in Nulliparous Obese Women' *American Journal of Obstetrics & Gynecology*, 200/4 (2009) 395.e1-9

210 P.S. Kaiser, R. S. Kirby 'Obesity as a Risk Factor for Cesarean in a Low-Risk Population' *Obstetrics & Gynecology* 97/1 (2001) 39-43

211 D. Rajasingam, P. T. Seed, A. L Briley et al, 'A Prospective Study of Pregnancy Outcome and Biomarkers of Oxidative Stress in Nulliparous Obese Women' *American Journal of Obstetrics & Gynecology*, 200/4 (2009) 395.e1-9

212 A. S. Poobalan, L. S. Aucott, T. Gurung et al 'Obesity as an Independent Risk Factor for Elective and Emergency Caesarean Delivery in Nulliparous Women - Systematic Review and Meta-Analysis of Cohort Studies' *Obesity Reviews*, 10/1 (2009) 28-35(8)

213 N. Schneid-Kofmana, E. Sheinera, A. Levyb et al 'Risk Factors for Wound Infection Following Cesarean Deliveries' *International Journal of Gynecology Obstetrics*, 90/1 (2004) 10-15

214 A. Caughey, N. Stotland, A. Washington et al 'Maternal Ethnicity, Paternal Ethnicity and Parental Ethnic Discordance: Predictors of Pre-Eclampsia' *Obstetrics & Gynecology*, 106/1 (2005) 156-61

215 NIH 'NIH State-of-the-Science Conference Statement on Cesarean Delivery on Maternal Request' *NIH Consensus State of the Science Statements* 23/1 (2006) 1-29

216 G. L. Gossman, J. M. Joesch, K. Tanfer K 'Trends in Maternal Request Cesarean Delivery from 1991 to 2004' *Obstetrics & Gynaecology*, 108/6 (2006) 1506-1516

217 J. Thomas, S. Paranjothy and Royal College of Obstetricians and Gynaecologists Clinical Effectiveness Support Unit. *National sentinel caesarean section audit report.* (London: RCOG Press, 2001)

218 J. Weaver, H. Statham, 'Wanting a caesarean section: the decision process' *BMJ*, 13/6 (2005) 1-5

219 C. McCourt, J. Weaver, H. Statham et al 'Elective Cesarean Section and Decision Making: A Critical Review of the Literature' *Birth*, 34/1 (2007) 65-79

220 J. Zhang, Y. Liu, S. Meikle et al 'Cesarean Delivery on Maternal Request in Southeast China' *Obstetrics & Gynecology*, 111/5 (2008) 1077-1082

221 J. A. Gamble, D. K. Creedy, 'Women's Preference for a Cesarean Section: Incidence and Associated Factors' *Birth* 28/2 (2001) 101-10

222 J. Weaver, H. Statham, M. Richards, 'A Study of Choice And Decision Making in Caesarean Section' *Report for Centre for Family Research,* University of Cambridge, (2002)

223 K. Hofberg, M. R. Ward, 'Fear Of Pregnancy And Childbirth' *Postgraduate Medical Journal* 79 (2003) 505-510

224 B. Areskog, N. Uddenberg, B. Kjessler 'Fear of Childbirth in Late Pregnancy' *Gynecologic &Obstetric Investigation* 12/5 (1981) 262-6

225 M. Laursen, M. Hedegaard, C. Johansen, 'Fear of Childbirth: Predictors and Temporal Changes Among Nulliparous Women in the Danish National Birth Cohort' *BJOG* 115/3 (2008) 354-60

226 J. Weaver, H. Statham, 'Wanting a caesarean section: the decision process' *BMJ* 13/6 (2005) 1-5

227 J. Green, H. Baston, S. Easton, 'Greater Expectations? Inter-Relationships Between Women's Expectations And Experiences of Decision Making, Continuity, Choice and Control in Labour, and Psychological Outcomes: Summary Report' *Leeds: Mother & Infant Research Unit* (2003)

228 J. Weaver, H. Statham, 'Wanting a caesarean section: the decision process' *BMJ* 13/6 (2005) 1-5

229 J. Fenwick, Y. Hauck, J. Downie et al, 'The Childbirth Expectations of a Self-Selected Cohort of Western Australian Women' *Midwifery,* 21/1 (2005) 23-35

230 J. Weaver, H. Statham, M. Richards, 'A Study of Choice And Decision Making in Caesarean Section' *Report for Centre for Family Research,* University of Cambridge, (2002)

231 K. Hofberg, M. R. Ward, 'Fear Of Pregnancy And Childbirth' *Postgraduate Medical Journal* 79 (2003) 505-510

232 H. Nerum, L. Halvorsen, T. Sørlie et al 'Maternal Request for Cesarean Section Due to Fear of Birth: Can it be Changed Through Crisis-Oriented Counseling?' *Birth,* 33/3 (2006) 221-8

233 B. Sjogren, 'Reasons for Anxiety About Childbirth in 100 Pregnant Women' *Journal of Psychosomatic Obstetrics & Gynecology* 18 (1997) 266-72

234 K. Hofberg, M. R. Ward, 'Fear Of Pregnancy And Childbirth' *Postgraduate Medical Journal* 79 (2003) 505-510

235 K. Hofberg, M. R. Ward, 'Fear Of Pregnancy And Childbirth' *Postgraduate Medical Journal* 79 (2003) 505-510

236 K Hofberg, 'Tokophobia: An Unreasoning Dread of Childbirth' *British Journal of Psychiatry* 176 (2000) 83-85

237 K. Wijma, J. Soderquist, B. Wijma, 'Posttraumatic Stress Disorder After Childbirth: A Cross Sectional Study' *Journal of Anxiety Disorders* 11/6 (1997) 587-97

238 E. L. Ryding, B. Wijma, K. Wijma, 'Posttraumatic Stress Reactions After Emergency Cesarean Section' *Acta Obstetrica Gynecologica Scandanavica,* 76/9 (1997) 856-61

239 R.E. Davis-Floyd 'The Technocratic Body: American Childbirth as Cultural Expression' *Social Science & Medicine,* 38/8 (1994) 1125-1140

240 J. Lally, M. Murtagh, S. Macphail et al, 'More in Hope Than Expectation: A Systematic Review of Women's Expectations and Experience of Pain Relief in Labour' *BMC Medicine,* (2008) 6:7doi:10.1186/1741-7015-6-7

241 R. Bakshi, A. Mehta, A. Mehta et al, 'Tokophobia: Fear Of Pregnancy And Childbirth' *The Internet Journal of Gynecology and Obstetrics,* 10/1 (2008)

242 C. Eriksson, L. Jansson, K. Hamberg, 'Women's Experiences of Intense Fear Related to Childbirth Investigated in a Swedish Qualitative Study' *Midwifery,* 22/3 (2006) 240-8

243 E. L. Ryding, 'Investigation of 33 Women Who Demanded A Cesarean Section For Personal Reasons' *Acta Obstetrica Gynecologica Scandanavica,* 72/4 (1993) 280-5

244 K Hofberg, 'Tokophobia: An Unreasoning Dread of Childbirth' *British Journal of Psychiatry* 176 (2000) 83-85

245 H. C. Lin, S. Xirasagar, 'Maternal Age and the Likelihood of a Maternal Request for Cesarean Delivery: A 5-Year Population-Based Study' *American Journal of Obstetrics and Gynachology* 192 (2005) 848-55

246 M.B. Landon, J. C. Hauth, K. J. Leveno et al, 'Maternal and Perinatal Outcomes Associated with a Trial of Labor after Prior Cesarean Delivery' *New England Journal of Medicine,* 351 (2004) 2581-2589

247 S. Paterson-Brown, 'Should Doctors Perform an Elective Caesarean Section on Request?' *BMJ* 317 (1998) 462

248 NICE, *Guideline for Caesarean Section,* (National Institute for Clinical Excellence, 2004)

249 European Collaborative Study 'Mother-to-child Transmission of HIV Infection in the Era of Highly Active Antiretroviral Therapy' *Clinical infectious diseases,* 40/3 (2005) 458-65

250 H. Nerum, L. Halvorsen, T. Sørlie et al 'Maternal Request for Cesarean Section Due to Fear of Birth: Can it be Changed Through Crisis-Oriented Counseling?' *Birth,* 33/3 (2006) 221-8

251 E. Banks, O. Meirik, T. Farley et al 'Female Genital Mutilation and Obstetric Outcome: WHO Collaborative Prospective Study in Six African Countries' *Lancet,* 367/9525 (2006) 1835-41

252 M. Connolly, D. Sullivan, *The Essential C-section Guide* (Broadway Books, 2004)

253 G. Barrett, J. Peacock, I Manyonda, 'Caesareans: a Short-Lived Honeymoon, Says Study into Sexual Function' *Brunel University and St George's Healthcare NHS Trust Press Release* (2006)

254 A. H. Sultan, M. A. Kamm, C. N. Hudson et al 'Anal-Sphincter Disruption During Vaginal Delivery' *New England Journal of Medicine,* 329/26 (1993) 1905-11

255 C. Larsson, K. Kallen, E. Andolf, 'Cesarean Section and Risk of Pelvic Organ Prolapse: A Nested Case-Control Study' *American Journal of Obstetrics and Gynaecology,* 200/3 (2009) 243.e1-4

256 S.C. Chua, S.J. Joung, R. Aziz, 'Incidence and Risk Factors Predicting Blood Transfusion in Caesarean Section' *Australian & New Zealand Journal of Obstetrics and Gynecology,* 49/5 (2009) 490-3

257 Childbirth.org 'Risk of caesarean section' *Childbirth.org* [on-line article] 1994 - accessed March 2011 < http://www.childbirth.org/section/risks.html>

258 M. Knight, J.J. Kurinczuk, P. Spark et al, 'Cesarean Delivery and Peripartum Hysterectomy' *Obstetric and Gynecology,* 111/1 (2008) 97-105

259 S.C. Chua, S.J. Joung, R. Aziz, 'Incidence and Risk Factors Predicting Blood Transfusion in Caesarean Section' *Australian & New Zealand Journal of Obstetrics and Gynecology*, 49/5 (2009) 490-3

260 M. Moore, C. de Costa, *Cesarean Section: Understanding and Celebrating Your Baby's Birth* (John Hopkins University Press, 2003)

261 M. Moore, C. de Costa, *Cesarean Section: Understanding and Celebrating Your Baby's Birth* (John Hopkins University Press, 2003)

262 RCOG, *Caesarean Section - Consent Advice No. 7,* (RCOG, 2009)

263 NICE, *Guideline for Caesarean Section,* (National Institute for Clinical Excellence, 2004)

264 M. Sandelowski, R. Bustamante, 'Cesarean Birth Outside the Natural Childbirth Culture' *Research in Nursing and Health* 9/2 (1986) 81-8

265 A. Tuteur, 'Who benefits from natural childbirth?' *The Skeptical OB* [on-line article] 2008 – accessed March 2010, <http://open.salon.com/blog/amytuteurmd/2008/08/27/who_benefits_from_natural_childbirth>

266 NICE, *Guideline for Caesarean Section,* (National Institute for Clinical Excellence, 2004)

267 RCOG, *Caesarean Section - Consent Advice No. 7,* (RCOG, 2009)

268 J. Fisher, J. Astbury, A. Smith, 'Adverse Psychological Impact Of Operative Obstetric Interventions: A Prospective Study' *Australian and New Zealand Journal of Psychiatry* 31/5 (1997) 728-738

269 Childbirth Connection, *What every pregnant woman needs to know about caesarean section,* (Childbirth Connection - 2nd Revised Edition, 2006)

270 M. Treadwell, 'Women Choosing Caesarean Have Low Death Rate' *Birth Trauma Association* [Press release] Oct 2008

271 CEMACH, 'Saving Mothers Lives – 2003-2005' *Confidential Enquiry into Maternal and Child Health* (2007) The Seventh Report of the Confidential Enquiries into Maternal Deaths in the United Kingdom

272 M. Treadwell, 'Women Choosing Caesarean Have Low Death Rate' *Birth Trauma Association* [Press release] Oct 2008

273 M. Connolly, D. Sullivan, *The Essential C-section Guide* (Broadway Books, 2004)

274 NHS, *NHS Maternity Statistics 2008-9,* (NHS Information Centre, Dec 2009).

275 Childbirth Connection, *What every pregnant woman needs to know about caesarean section,* (Childbirth Connection - 2nd Revised Edition, 2006)

276 NHS, *Latest Maternity Statistics Show How the Pattern of Giving Birth in England is Changing,* (NHS Information Centre, 2008)

277 NHS, *NHS Maternity Statistics 2008-9,* (NHS Information Centre, Dec 2009).

278 J. Green, H. Baston, S. Easton, 'Greater Expectations? Inter-Relationships Between Women's Expectations And Experiences of Decision Making, Continuity, Choice and Control in Labour, and Psychological Outcomes: Summary Report' *Leeds: Mother & Infant Research Unit* (2003)

279 S. Paterson-Brown, 'Elective Caesarean Section: A Woman's Right to Choose?' *Progress in Obstetrics and Gynaecology* J Studd, Ed. (2000)14:202-15

280 M. Enkin, M. Keirse, J. Neilson et al *A Guide to Effective Care in Pregnancy and Childbirth* (Oxford University Press, 2000), Chapter 41 - 'Instrumental Vaginal Delivery'

281 S.A. Farrell, 'Cesarean Section Versus Forceps Assisted Vaginal Birth: It's Time to Include Pelvic Injury in the Risk–Benefit Equation' *CMAJ*, 166/3 (2002)

282 NHS, *NHS Maternity Statistics 2007-8*, NHS Information Centre, 2009

283 RCOG, *A Third or Fourth-Degree Tear During Childbirth: Information For You*, (RCOG, 2008)

284 B. Lane, 'Epidural Rates in the US and Around the World: How Many Mothers Choose to Use an Epidural to Provide Pain Relief?' *Suite101.com* [on-line article] Nov. 2009 – accessed August 2010 , http://www.suite101.com/content/epidural-for-labor-a168170>

285 E. Declercq, C. Sakala, M. Corry, et al, 'Listening to Mothers: Report of the First National U.S. Survey of Women's Childbearing Experiences' *Maternity Centre Association*, [on-line report], Oct. 2002 - accessed March 2011
< http://www.childbirthconnection.org/pdfs/LtMreport.pdf>

286 NHS, *NHS Maternity Statistics 2008-9*, (NHS Information Centre, Dec 2009).

287 J.M. Guise, K. Eden, C. Emeis et al, 'Vaginal Birth After Cesarean: New Insights. Evidence Report/Technology Assessment No.191.' *Oregon Health & Science University Evidence-based Practice Center (*2010)

288 S.I. Kayani, Z. Alfirevic. 'Uterine Rupture After Induction of Labour in Women With Previous Caesarean Section' *BJOG*, 112/4 (2005) 451-5

289 RCOG, *Birth After Previous Caesarean*, (RCOG, 2008)

290 NICE, *Guideline for Caesarean Section*, (National Institute for Clinical Excellence, 2004)

291 D. Chippington-Derrick, G. Lowdon, F. Barlow *Caesarean Birth - Your Questions Answered*, (NCT Publication, 2004)

292 J.M. Guise, K. Eden, C. Emeis et al, 'Vaginal Birth After Cesarean: New Insights. Evidence Report/Technology Assessment No.191.' *Oregon Health & Science University Evidence-based Practice Center (*2010)

293 G.C. Smith, J.P. Pell, A.D. Cameron et al, 'Risk of Perinatal Death Associated with Labor After Previous Caesarean Delivery in Uncomplicated Term Pregnancies' *JAMA*, 287/20 (2002) 2684-90

294 D. Levin, 'Pregnancy Complications: Uterine Rupture' *Healthline.com* [on-line article] 2006 – accessed Aug 2010
<http://www.healthline.com/yodocontent/pregnancy/complications-uterine-rupture.html>

295 G.G. Nahum, K.Q. Pham, 'Uterine Rupture in Pregnancy' *emedicine.medscape.com* [on-line article] May 2010 - accessed Aug 2010 < http://emedicine.medscape.com/article/275854-overview>

296 NICE, *Guideline for Caesarean Section*, (National Institute for Clinical Excellence, 2004)

297 RCOG, *A Third or Fourth-Degree Tear During Childbirth: Information For You*, (RCOG, 2008)

298 E. Declercq, C. Sakala, M. Corry, et al, 'Listening to Mothers: Report of the First National U.S. Survey of Women's Childbearing Experiences' *Maternity Centre Association*, [on-line

report], Oct. 2002 - accessed March 2011
< http://www.childbirthconnection.org/pdfs/LtMreport.pdf>

299 M. Treadwell, 'Women Choosing Caesarean Have Low Death Rate' *Birth Trauma Association* [Press release] Oct 2008

300 CEMACH, 'Saving Mothers Lives – 2003-2005' *Confidential Enquiry into Maternal and Child Health* (2007) The Seventh Report of the Confidential Enquiries into Maternal Deaths in the United Kingdom

301 CEMACH, 'Saving Mothers Lives – 2003-2005' *Confidential Enquiry into Maternal and Child Health* (2007) The Seventh Report of the Confidential Enquiries into Maternal Deaths in the United Kingdom

302 B. Ashcroft, M. Elstein, N. Boreham et al 'Prospective Semi-Structured Observational Study to Identify Risk Attributable to Staff Deployment, Training, and Updating Opportunities for Midwives' *BMJ* 327/584 (2003)

303 J. Thomas, S. Paranjothy and Royal College of Obstetricians and Gynaecologists Clinical Effectiveness Support Unit. *National sentinel caesarean section audit report.* (London: RCOG Press, 2001)

304 R. Pelling, 'If You are Thinking of Giving Birth in Britain, Listen to This', *The Independent On-line*, 30 January 2005

305 M. Enkin, M. Keirse, J. Neilson et al *A Guide to Effective Care in Pregnancy and Childbirth* (Oxford University Press, 2000), Chapter 28 - 'Social and Professional Support in Childbirth'

306 J.M. Alexander, K.J. Leveno, J. Hauth et al 'Fetal Injury Associated With Cesarean Delivery' *Obstetrics & Gynecology*, 108/4 (2006) 885-90

307 J.M. Alexander, K.J. Leveno, J. Hauth et al 'Fetal Injury Associated With Cesarean Delivery' *Obstetrics & Gynecology*, 108/4 (2006) 885-90

308 D.M. Haas, A.W. Ayres 'Laceration Injury at Cesarean Delivery' *Journal Maternal Fetal & Neonatal Medicine*, 11/3 (2002) 196-8.

309 A. Kirkeby Hansen, K. Wisborg, N. Uldbjerg et al, 'Risk of Respiratory Morbidity in Term Infants Delivered by Elective Caesarean Section: Cohort Study' *BMJ* doi:10 1136/bmj.39405.539282.BE (2007)

310 NIH 'NIH State-of-the-Science Conference Statement on Cesarean Delivery on Maternal Request' *NIH Consensus State of the Science Statements* 23/1 (2006) 1–29

311 NICE, *Guideline for Caesarean Section*, (National Institute for Clinical Excellence, 2004)

312 A.E. Nicoll, C. Black, A. Powls et al 'An Audit of Neonatal Respiratory Morbidity Following Elective Caesarean Section at Term' *Scottish Medical Journal* 49/1 (2004) 22-25

313 UAB.edu 'Study Shows Risk to Babies in Elective Early Term Csections' *UAB.edu* [Press Release] 2009 – accessed Aug 2010 <http://main.uab.edu/Sites/reporter/articles/57111/>

314 J.J. Morrison, J.M. Rennie, P.J. Milton, 'Neonatal Respiratory Morbidity and Mode of Delivery at Term: Influence of Timing of Elective Caesarean Section' *BJOG* 102 (1995) 101-10

315 A. Kirkeby Hansen, K. Wisborg, N. Uldbjerg et al, 'Risk of Respiratory Morbidity in Term Infants Delivered by Elective Caesarean Section: Cohort Study' *BMJ* doi:10 1136/bmj.39405.539282.BE (2007)

316 J. Madar, S. Richmond, E. Hey, 'Surfactant-Deficient Respiratory Distress after Elective Delivery at Term' *Acta Paediatrica* 88/11 (1999) 1244-1248

317 H.J. Rowe-Murray, J.R. Fisher, 'Baby Friendly Hospital Practices: Cesarean Section is a Persistent Barrier to Early Initiation of Breastfeeding' *Birth*, 29/2 (2002) 124-31

318 A. Maitra, A. Sherriff, D. Strachan et al J 'Mode of Delivery is Not Associated with Asthma or Atopy in Childhood' *Clinical and Experimental Allergy* 34/9 (2004) 1349-55

319 Y.J. Juhn, A. Weaver, S. Katusic et al 'Mode of Delivery at Birth and Development of Asthma: A Population-Based Cohort Study' *Journal of Allergy and Clinical Immunology* 116/3 (2005) 510-6

320 J.S. Debley, J.M. Smith, G.J. Redding et al, 'Childhood Asthma Hospitalization Risk after Cesarean Delivery in Former Term and Premature Infants' *Annals of Allergy, Asthma & Immunology*, 94/2 (2005) 228-33

321 C. Roduit, S. Scholtens, J.C. de Jongste et al 'Asthma at 8 Years of Age in Children Born by Caesarean Section' *Thorax* 64:107-113 doi:10.1136/thx.2008.100875 (2009)

322 G.C.S. Smith, A.M. Wood, I.R. White et al, 'Neonatal Respiratory Morbidity at Term and the Risk of Childhood Asthma' *Archives of Disease in Childhood* 89 (2004) 956-960

323 T. Kolas, O. Saugstad, A. Daltveit et al, 'Planned Cesarean Versus Planned Vaginal Delivery at Term: Comparison of Newborn Infant Outcomes' *American Journal of Obstetrics and Gynecology* 195 (2006) 1538-43

324 M. Moore, C. de Costa, *Cesarean Section: Understanding and Celebrating Your Baby's Birth* (John Hopkins University Press, 2003)

325 NICE, *Guideline for Caesarean Section*, (National Institute for Clinical Excellence, 2004)

326 M. Enkin, M. Keirse, J. Neilson et al *A Guide to Effective Care in Pregnancy and Childbirth* (Oxford University Press, 2000), Chapter 41 - 'Instrumental Vaginal Delivery'

327 R.S. Galbraith, 'Incidence of Neonatal Sixth Nerve Palsy in Relation to Mode of Delivery' *American Journal of Obstetrics and Gynecology*, 170/4 (1994) 1158-9

328 RCOG, *A Difficult Birth: What is Shoulder Dystocia?* (RCOG, 2007)

329 D. Towner, M.A. Castro, E. Eby-Wilkens et al, 'Effect of Mode of Delivery in Nulliparous Women on Neonatal Intracranial Injury' *New England Journal of Medicine* 341/23 (1999) 1709-14

330 NICE, *Guideline for Caesarean Section*, (National Institute for Clinical Excellence, 2004)

331 NHS, *Latest Maternity Statistics Show How the Pattern of Giving Birth in England is Changing*, (NHS Information Centre, 2008)

332 P. Millns, K. Eagland K *Anaesthesia and Having a Baby* (Birmingham Women's Hospital publication u.d)

333 D. Chippington-Derrick, G. Lowdon, F. Barlow *Caesarean Birth – Your Questions Answered*, (NCT Publication, 2004)

334 OAA *Your Anaesthetic for Caesarean Section*, (Obstetric Anaesthetists' Association, 2009)

335 OAA *Your Anaesthetic for Caesarean Section*, (Obstetric Anaesthetists' Association, 2009)

336 OAA *Your Anaesthetic for Caesarean Section*, (Obstetric Anaesthetists' Association, 2009)

337 L. Smith 'Fears over risk of having an epidural exaggerated' *The Sunday Times* [on-line article] 2009 – accessed Aug 2010
<http://www.timesonline.co.uk/tol/life_and_style/health/article5497517.ece>

338 OAA *Your Anaesthetic for Caesarean Section,* (Obstetric Anaesthetists' Association, 2009)

339 OAA *Your Anaesthetic for Caesarean Section,* (Obstetric Anaesthetists' Association, 2009)

340 OAA *Your Anaesthetic for Caesarean Section,* (Obstetric Anaesthetists' Association, 2009)

341 RCOA, *Risks Associated With your Anaesthetic: Section 8 - Awareness During Anaesthesia* (Royal College of Anaesthetists , 2010)

342 R.J. Pollard, J.P. Coyle, R.L. Gilbert et al, 'Intraoperative Awareness in a Regional Medical System: A Review of 3 Years' Data' *Anesthesiology,* 106/2 (2007) 269-74

343 OAA *Your Anaesthetic for Caesarean Section,* (Obstetric Anaesthetists' Association, 2009)

344 OAA *Your Anaesthetic for Caesarean Section,* (Obstetric Anaesthetists' Association, 2009)

345 OAA *Your Anaesthetic for Caesarean Section,* (Obstetric Anaesthetists' Association, 2009)

346 OAA *Your Anaesthetic for Caesarean Section,* (Obstetric Anaesthetists' Association, 2009)

347 RCOG, *Caesarean Section - Consent Advice No. 7,* (RCOG, 2009)

348 N. Tharpe, 'Postpregnancy Genital Tract and Wound Infections' *Journal of Midwifery & Women's Health,* 53/3 (2008) 236-246

349 Childbirth Connection, *What every pregnant woman needs to know about caesarean section,* (Childbirth Connection - 2nd Revised Edition, 2006)

350 K.G. Dewey, 'Maternal and Fetal Stress Are Associated with Impaired Lactogenesis in Humans' *Journal of Nutrition,* 131 (2001) 3012-3015

351 R. Grajeda, R. Pérez-Escamilla. 'Stress During Labor and Delivery Is Associated with Delayed Onset of Lactation among Urban Guatemalan Women'*Journal of Nutrition,* 132 (2002) 3055-60

352 C. Tatano Beck, S. Watson, 'Impact of Birth Trauma on Breastfeeding: A Tale of Two Pathways' *Nursing Research,* 57/4 (2007) 228-236

353 Childbirth Connection, *What every pregnant woman needs to know about caesarean section,* (Childbirth Connection - 2nd Revised Edition, 2006)

354 J. Jolly, J. Walker, K. Bhabra, 'Subsequent Obstetric Performance Related to Primary Mode of Delivery' *BJOG* 106: 227–232. doi: 10.1111/j.1471-0528.1999.tb08235.x (2005)

355 J. Green, H. Baston, S. Easton, 'Greater Expectations? Inter-Relationships Between Women's Expectations And Experiences of Decision Making, Continuity, Choice and Control in Labour, and Psychological Outcomes: Summary Report' *Leeds: Mother & Infant Research Unit* (2003)

356 J. Green, H. Baston, S. Easton, 'Greater Expectations? Inter-Relationships Between Women's Expectations And Experiences of Decision Making, Continuity, Choice and Control in Labour, and Psychological Outcomes: Summary Report' *Leeds: Mother & Infant Research Unit* (2003)

357 J. Lally, M. Murtagh, S. Macphail et al, 'More in Hope Than Expectation: A Systematic Review of Women's Expectations and Experience of Pain Relief in Labour' *BMC Medicine* (2008) 6:7doi:10.1186/1741-7015-6-7

358 M. Connolly, D. Sullivan, *The Essential C-section Guide* (Broadway Books, 2004)

359 G. Barrett, J. Peacock, I Manyonda, 'Caesareans: a Short-Lived Honeymoon, Says Study into Sexual Function' *Brunel University and St George's Healthcare NHS Trust Press Release* (2006)

360 N. Tharpe, 'Postpregnancy Genital Tract and Wound Infections' *Journal of Midwifery & Women's Health,* 53/3 (2008) 236-246

361 C.V. Ananth, J.C. Smulian, A.M. Vintzileos, 'The Association of Placenta Previa with History of Caesarean Delivery and Abortion: A Meta-analysis' *American journal of Obstetrics and Gynecology,* 177/5 (1997)

362 M. Connolly, D. Sullivan, *The Essential C-section Guide* (Broadway Books, 2004)

363 G. Dildy, 'Last 50 Years Show 10-fold Rise in Placenta Accreta – Behind 50% of Emergency Hysterectomies ', *The Free Library* [on-line article] u.d – accessed Aug 2010

364 Patient.co.uk 'Antepartum Haemorrhage' *Patient.co.uk* [on-line article] Feb. 2011 - accessed March 2011 < http://www.patient.co.uk/doctor/Antepartum-Haemorrhage.htm>

365 G. Dildy, 'Last 50 Years Show 10-fold Rise in Placenta Accreta – Behind 50% of Emergency Hysterectomies ', *The Free Library* [on-line article] u.d – accessed Aug 2010

366 M. Connolly, D. Sullivan, *The Essential C-section Guide* (Broadway Books, 2004)

367 M. Connolly, D. Sullivan, *The Essential C-section Guide* (Broadway Books, 2004)

368 D.J. Murphy, G.M. Stirrat, J. Heron, 'The Relationship Between Caesarean Section and Sub Fertility in a Population-Based Sample of 14,541 Pregnancies' *Journal of Human Reproduction,* 17/7 (2002) 1914-1917

369 E. Hemminki, H.J. Hoffman, B.I. Graubard et al, 'Cesarean Section and Subsequent Fertility: Results from the 1982 National Survey of Family Growth' *Fertility and Sterility,* 43 (1985) 520-528

370 J. Mollison, M. Porter, D. Campbell et al, 'Primary Mode of Delivery and Subsequent Pregnancy' *BJOG,* 112/8 (2005) 1061-65

371 J. Mollison, M. Porter, D. Campbell et al, 'Primary Mode of Delivery and Subsequent Pregnancy' *BJOG,* 112/8 (2005) 1061-65

372 L. Saraswat. M. Porter, S. Bhattacharya et al, 'Caesarean Section and Tubal Infertility: is there an Association?' *Reproductive Biomedicine Online* 17/2 (2008) 259-64

373 M.E. Wolf, J.R. Daling, L.F. Voigt, 'Prior Cesarean Delivery in Women with Secondary Tubal Infertility' *American Journal of Public Health,* 80 (1990) 1382-1383

374 D. Bider, J. Blankstein, I. Tur Kaspa, 'Fertility in Anovulatory Patients after Primary Cesarean Section' *Journal of Reproductive Medicine,* 43 (1998) 869-871

375 D.J. Murphy, G.M. Stirrat, J. Heron, 'The Relationship Between Caesarean Section and Sub Fertility in a Population-Based Sample of 14,541 Pregnancies' *Journal of Human Reproduction,* 17/7 (2002) 1914-1917

376 M. Porter, S. Bhattacharyal, E. van Teijlingen et al, 'Does Caesarean Section Cause Infertility?' *Human Reproduction,* 23/3 (2008) 543-547

377 K. Gottvall, U. Waldenstrom, 'Does a Traumatic Birth Experience Have an Impact on Future Reproduction?' *BJOG,* 109 (2002) 254-260

378 J. Jolly, J. Walker, K. Bhabra, 'Subsequent Obstetric Performance Related to Primary Mode of Delivery' *BJOG* 106: 227–232. doi: 10.1111/j.1471-0528.1999.tb08235.x (2005)

379 M.C. Tollanes, K.K. Melve, L.M. Irgens et al, 'Reduced Fertility after Caesarean Delivery: A Maternal Choice' Obstetrics and Gynachology 110 (6 (2007) 1256-63

380 K. Gottvall, U. Waldenstrom, 'Does a Traumatic Birth Experience Have an Impact on Future Reproduction?' *BJOG,* 109 (2002) 254–260

381 R. Bahl, B. Strachan, D.J. Murphy, 'Outcome of Subsequent Pregnancy Three Years after Previous Operative Delivery in the Second Stage of Labour: Cohort Study' *BMJ,* doi:10.1136/bmj.37942.546076.44 (2004)

382 M. Porter, S. Bhattacharyal, E. van Teijlingen et al, 'Does Caesarean Section Cause Infertility?' *Human Reproduction,* 23/3 (2008) 543-547

383 Childbirth Connection, *What every pregnant woman needs to know about caesarean section,* (Childbirth Connection - 2nd Revised Edition, 2006)

384 M. Connolly, D. Sullivan, *The Essential C-section Guide* (Broadway Books, 2004)

385 T. Shipp, C. Zelop, J. Repeke et al, 'Interdelivery Interval and Risk of Symptomatic Uterine Rupture' *Obstetrics and Gynecology,* 97/2 (2001) 175-7

386 E. Bujold, S.H. Mehta, C. Bujold et al, 'Interdelivery Interval and Uterine Rupture' *American Journal of Obstetrics and Gynecology* 187/5 (2002) 1199-202

387 NICE, *Guideline for Caesarean Section,* (National Institute for Clinical Excellence, 2004)

388 NICE, *Guideline for Caesarean Section,* (National Institute for Clinical Excellence, 2004)

389RCOG, *Birth After Previous Caesarean,* (RCOG, 2008)

390 NICE, *Guideline for Caesarean Section,* (National Institute for Clinical Excellence, 2004)

391 C.S. Cotzias, S. Paterson-Brown, N.M. Fisk, 'Prospective Risk of Unexplained Stillbirth in Singleton Pregnancies at Term: Population Based Analysis' *BMJ* 319/7205 (1999) 287–288

392 M. O. Bahtiyar, S. Julien, J. N. Robinson et al, 'Prior Cesarean Delivery is Not Associated with an Increased Risk of Stillbirth in a Subsequent Pregnancy: Analysis of U.S. Perinatal Mortality Data, 1995-1997' *American Journal of Obstetrics and Gynecology* 195/5 (2006) 1373-8

393 S.L. Wood, S. Chen, S. Ross et al, 'The Risk of Unexplained Antepartum Stillbirth in Second Pregnancies Following Caesarean Section in the First Pregnancy' *BJOG,* 115/6 (2008) 726-31

394 BBC News 'No stillbirth link' to Caesarean' *BBC News* [on-line article] 6th June 2008 – accessed Aug 2010 <http://news.bbc.co.uk/1/hi/health/7433884.stm>

395 R. Gray, M.A. Quigley, C. Hockley et al, 'Caesarean Delivery and Risk of Stillbirth in Subsequent Pregnancy: A Retrospective Cohort Study in an English Population' *BJOG,* 114/3 (2007) 264-70

396 Association for Postnatal Illness 'Postnatal Depression' *Association for Postnatal Illness* [on-line leaflet] u.d - accessed Aug 2010 <http://apni.org/Post-Natal-Deperession-Leaflet.html>

397 M. Moore, C. de Costa, *Cesarean Section: Understanding and Celebrating Your Baby's Birth* (John Hopkins University Press, 2003)

398 R. Patel, D. Murphy, T. Peters, 'Operative Delivery and Postnatal Depression: A Cohort Study' *BMJ* 330/7496 (2005) 879

399 Psychiatry Research Trust, 'Postnatal Depression' *Psychiatry Research Trust,* [on-line article] u.d. – accessed Aug 2010 <http://www.iop.kcl.ac.uk/iop/prt/pnd.htm>

400 S. Ayres, A.D. Pickering, 'Do Women get Posttraumatic Stress Disorder as A Result of Childbirth? A Prospective Study of Incidence' *Birth,* 28/2 (2001) 111-8

401 E. Olde, O. van der Hart, R. Kleber et al, 'Posttraumatic Stress Following Childbirth: A Review' *Clinical Psychology Review* 26/1 (2006) 1-16

402 J. Czarnocka, P. Slade, 'Prevelance and Predictors of Post-Traumatic Stress Symptoms Following Childbirth' *British Journal of Clinical Psychology,* 39/1 (2000) 35-51

403 J. Soderquist, K. Wijima, B. Wijima, 'Traumatic Stress in Late Pregnancy' *Journal of Anxiety Disorders* 18/2 (2004) 127-142

404 PANDA (Post and Antenatal Depression Association) 'Men and Postnatal Depression: How Postnatal Depression can Affect Fathers' *Raising Children Network* [on-line article] Jan. 2010 - accessed March 2010
<http://raisingchildren.net.au/articles/men_and_postnatal_depression.html>

405 E. Bielawska-Batorowicz, K. Kossakowska-Petrycka 'Depressive Mood in Men after the Birth of their Offspring in Relation to a Partner's Depression, Social Support, Fathers' Personality And Prenatal Expectations' *Journal of Reproductive and Infant Psychology,* 24/1 (2006) 21-29

406 PANDA (Post and Antenatal Depression Association) 'Men and Postnatal Depression: How Postnatal Depression can Affect Fathers' *Raising Children Network* [on-line article] Jan. 2010 - accessed March 2010
<http://raisingchildren.net.au/articles/men_and_postnatal_depression.html>

407 *Biology of Dads* (2010) BBC TV Production

408 J.F. Paulson, H.A. Keefe, J.A. Leiferman, 'Early Parental Depression and Child Language Development' *Journal of Child Psychology & Psychiatry* 50/3 (2009) 254-62

Index

CPSIA information can be obtained at www.ICGtesting.com
Printed in the USA
244582LV00009B/30/P